LEGAL MEDICINE 1987

LEGAL MEDICINE 1987

CYRIL H. WECHT,
M.D., J.D., Series Editor

Former Coroner, Allegheny County (Pittsburgh), Pa.; Clinical Adjunct Professor of Pathology, University of Pittsburgh Schools of Medicine and Dental Medicine; Adjunct Associate Professor of Epidemiology, University of Pittsburgh Graduate School of Public Health; Adjunct Professor of Pathology and Legal Medicine, Duquesne University School of Pharmacy; Adjunct Professor of Law, Duquesne University School of Law; Director, Pittsburgh Institute of Legal Medicine; Past President, American Academy of Forensic Sciences; Past President, American College of Legal Medicine.

PRAEGER

New York
Westport, Connecticut
London

ISBN: 0–275–92595–1
ISSN: 0197–9981
Library of Congress Catalog Card Number: 80–647751

Library of Congress Catalog Card Number: 80–647751
ISBN: 0–275–92595–1
ISSN: 0197–9981

First published in 1988

Praeger Publishers, One Madison Avenue, New York, NY 10010
A division of Greenwood Press, Inc.

The paper used in this book complies with the
Permanent Paper Standard issued by the National
Information Standards Organization (Z39.48–1984).

10 9 8 7 6 5 4 3 2 1

Contents

Contributors

A. Bernard Ackerman, M.D. Professor of Dermatology and Pathology, and Director of Dermatopathology, New York University School of Medicine, New York, New York

Sharon M. Camissa, Esquire. Public Defender's Office, Solano County, Fairfield, California

James B. Couch, M.D., J.D., F.C.L.M. Director of Health and Medical Systems, Hahnemann University, Philadelphia, Pennsylvania

Francis M. Esposito, Ph.D. Associate Toxicologist, Allegheny County Department of Laboratories, Pittsburgh, Pennsylvania

Bernard J. Ficarra, M.D., Sc.D., Ph.D., LL.D., J.D. Member, Professional Editorial Board, *Journal of Contemporary Health, Law and Policy*, The Catholic University of America Law School, Washington, D.C.

Marvin S. Fish, Esquire. Partner, Law Firm of Slavitt, Fish & Cowen, P.A., Newark, New Jersey

Nathaniel Shafer, M.D. Assistant Clinical Professor, New York Medical College, New York, New York

Douglas R. Shanklin, A.B., M.D. Professor of Pathology and of Obstetrics and Gynecology, University of Tennessee College of Medicine, Memphis, Tennessee

Richard Arnold Silver, M.D. Medical Director, Sports Medicine Clinic of Tucson, Tucson, Arizona

Cyril H. Wecht, M.D., J.D. Clinical Associate Professor of Pathology, University of Pittsburgh Schools of Medicine and Dental Medicine, Pittsburgh, Pennsylvania

Charles L. Winek, Ph.D. Director and Chief Toxicologist, Allegheny County Department of Laboratories, Pittsburgh, Pennsylvania

Natalie Ziontz, Esquire. Member of the Law Firm of Lewis, D'Amato, Brisbois & Bisgaard, Los Angeles, California

Preface

It is difficult to define the parameters of legal medicine because of its broad, varied, and ever-expanding societal ramifications; hence, it is quite a challenge to blend together chapters covering a sufficiently wide range of subjects that are uniformly enticing and informative with utilitarian value to civil and criminal trial attorneys, forensic scientists, physicians, and other health care personnel involved in medico-legal matters. *Legal Medicine 1987* is another volume in our continuing effort to reach out to all these professional groups with timely, substantive topics discussed by experienced, acknowledged experts.

The subjects deal with practical medical-legal needs and experiences that should provide useful information for our readers. All the chapters relate to subjects that are appropriate and highly desirable for inclusion within any academic legal medicine program. They also constitute a worthwhile compilation of authoritative reference materials for professional medical and legal libraries.

I am indebted to all the contributing authors for their valuable time and personal consideration. As in past years, the efforts of my personal secretary, Maribeth Blettner, have been invaluable in organizing and editing this book.

Cyril H. Wecht

LEGAL MEDICINE 1987

1. Private Consulting Forensic Pathology

Douglas R. Shanklin, A.B., M.D.

Sir Arthur Conan Doyle, in his brilliant first novel concerning Sherlock Holmes, *A Study in Scarlet*, illustrates with precise clarity the role of a private investigator of crime[12]. The preliminaries of the conversation between John H. Watson, M.D., and Mr. Holmes have ended, and the two turn their attention to a message sent by Inspector Tobias Gregson of Scotland Yard that asks Mr. Holmes to come to Lauriston Gardens to aid in the investigation of the death of one Enoch J. Drebber of Cleveland, Ohio. This will eventually set into motion the entire, convoluted plot which, as most readers know well, will range from the Sierra Blancos and the Great Alkali Plain of the American West to the byways of London. Initially, however, Holmes is Hamlet-like in his reaction to the invitation, hesitating before this obvious opportunity even as his newfound friend urges him on. Then, Doyle has Holmes explain his hesitancy role in a very succinct manner: "That comes of being an unofficial personage[12]." And thus it is for the private consulting forensic pathologist.

The past twenty years have seen a continuing discussion in the medical literature on medicolegal investigating systems and on forensic pathology[1,2,4–11,14,16,18–22,30,31,34,35]. Interestingly, much of this commentary is to be found in the pages of the leading general medical journal in the U.S., *The New England Journal of Medicine*. Labelled the "invisible profession" by James L. Luke[20], forensic pathology became very visible to the public at large during the long run of the popular television show, "Quincy, M.E.," starring Jack Klugman.

Undoubtedly, the program performed a valuable public service in illustrating the degree of sophistication the forensic sciences have reached in general. The major failing in the program, however, was its poor sense of time. This could have been helped, even in a one-hour program, by the occasional use of a line like, "You'll have such and such by next Tuesday." Nonetheless, what the show rarely got away from—and it could not do so very often, given its basic format and physical location—was its presentation of forensic pathology merely as a branch of the police investigative function and the prosecutorial side of criminal law. Only a few episodes involved death investigation in the civil realm or concerned the interests of the accused. The story of the athlete who collapsed from an ectopic functioning pheochromocytoma was a notable exception.

The aforementioned general discussion on forensic medicine included Corrigan's concept of forensic pathology as the *pathology of public health*[5], a construct extending the more commonly understood role of public health. To some extent, this function carried out nationally by the Center for Disease Control, albeit epidemiologically, and not in the case-specific, investigative manner suggested by Corrigan. Public health departments have generally enjoyed the reputation of and acted as genuinely independent agencies with some direct powers of action or enforcement. Medical examiner's systems have been constructed in various ways in the several states. The author is most familiar with the evolution of the system in Florida, having worked in it off and on for a number of years as an assistant examiner and substitute district medical examiner, a total of twenty-two years of direct observation in one capacity or another, including that of "an unofficial personage." Florida statutes embody the tension of independent responsibility versus affiliation with law enforcement. F.S. 406.02[1] specifically defines a medical examiners' commission, the state oversight agency, as being "within the Department of Law Enforcement." However, F.S. 406.12 places an affirmative duty on "any person" to report *directly* (emphasis added) to the district medical examiner any death and the circumstances surrounding it from a comprehensive, generally standard list of forensic situations. Contrariwise, F.S. 406.13 requires the district medical examiner to report to the state attorney the findings as to the cause of death.

Florida has a modern system of district public defenders. These officials are not mentioned anywhere in the medical examiner statutes. Considered even less often are private defense attorneys or private consulting forensic pathologists. The nearly inevitable result of such arrangements is that these private consultants become part of the investigation when appropriate in the judicial system only following requests by various defense counsel *after* primary investigation and the filing of charges or indictment. As such, the unofficial personage, like Sherlock Holmes, becomes an expert in remote evidence and cold trails. Inference and deduction become stock-in-trade.

The following is an account of specific examples of forensic consultation in both criminal and civil proceedings, not always with express legal connotation. These accounts, drawn from the author's personal experience, are offered to demonstrate aspects of the present functioning of medical examiners' systems in the United States. Several have been reported earlier in greater detail, but in what can be called the *acta obscura*[27].

ACTING AS CONTRACT PATHOLOGIST

These cases were brought to the attention of the author by attorneys acting on behalf of their clients, or sometimes directly by the representatives of insurance companies.

Reinterpretation of Surgical Pathology

A man in his late fifties was experiencing some difficulty in urination. He consulted a urologist, who found prostatic enlargement and recommended transurethral resection. This was done soon after, and the pathology laboratory tentatively reported microscopic cancer. The slides were sent out for consultation, but the consultant was away for an extended period. After several weeks delay, the chief assistant to the consultant reported the case as confirmed for malignancy, and a radical prostatectomy was done. The second surgical specimen revealed no remnants of carcinoma. The patient had a difficult course and became impotent. Another clinician doubted the wisdom of the second procedure, and eventually the man consulted an attorney. The attorney came to the author. Neither I nor any of the more than twelve other pathologists to whom I showed the material could make a diagnosis of malignancy, although some glandular atypia was present. The eventual lawsuit was settled just prior to trial in favor of the plaintiff, who remained alive without any evidence of tumor over eight years after the primary procedure.

In this case, the contract pathologist served mainly as a resource person, providing entry to a wider range of consultative opinion than the avenue chosen by the initial hospital laboratory. The case does point up the occasional misdirection of consultative patterns. This has a general application beyond the needs of forensic pathology. It has been the experience of the author that these things are not well systematized either regionally or nationally. The future of institutional medicine, in particular as it relates to the marketing of services, may well come to have an influence on these needs. A fuller discussion of such problems is beyond the scope of this article.

Protection of Tissues Removed Surgically or at Postmortem

A 29-year-old man was contemplating his fourth open-heart procedure in eight years. An action had been filed earlier over events allegedly occurring during the second procedure. This operation involved replacement of an aortic valve prothesis put in five years earlier plus replacement of late-stage rheumatic mitral valve disease with a prosthetic valve. Persistent heart failure after the second operation prompted a third some four months later. During that procedure, two sutures were found to have come apart, either from product failure or from inadvertent cutting part way through during placement. The patient's attorney requested a court order to preserve as evidence any tissue removed during the fourth operation. The author was appointed as conservator in place of the hospital's department of pathology. The surgeon was most co-operative, and when he found he had to remove the prosthesis placed some three years earlier, he called me and the device was placed in my custody. The multiple procedures had taken their toll, however, and further attempts to strengthen the heart surgically a month later failed. Still acting as conservator, the author participated in the autopsy, filing a report with the executor of the estate. Recently, the original action went to trial, but despite there being no evidence of a third alternative, the jury found neither the original surgeons nor the suture manufacturer liable for the failure of the two sutures. They were adjacent on the original mitral sewing ring and a significant leak had occurred around the prosthesis at that point.

In this case, the contract pathologist became a personal representative of a patient, acting under court order, and made primary observations both on surgically removed tissue and at autopsy, even though he was not a member of the staff of the hospital at which these procedures were done. Study of the removed primary mitral prosthesis did have a bearing on interpretation of the events of three years earlier and, thus, on the cause of death.

Reinterpretation of Autopsy Pathology

A 17-year-old black man sustained leg injuries treated by intramedullary nailing of both femurs. A year later he underwent spinal anesthesia for removal of hardware but sustained respiratory arrest; immediate cardiopulmonary resuscitation was successful but the patient remained unresponsive and died a few days later. Autopsy permission was obtained, but during the actual performance of the postmortem the family withdrew permission. The family prevailed upon the district medical examiner to convert the case to his jurisdiction. A second autopsy was then done on the body although the first one was not fully completed at time of transfer. Despite a double autopsy, no fully satisfactory cause of death was determined. Both sets of tissue slides and the complete files were sent to the author by an attorney acting for the family. It was immediately obvious that the cause of death was sickle cell crisis. Impactions were found in eleven different organs, along with marked pulmonary edema. The young man resembled his father more than he did his mother, particularly in his rather prominent supraorbital ridges. This fact was of importance because hemoglobin electrophoresis showed the father to be SA and the mother AA. No sickle cell testing of any kind had been done on the young man.

In this case the contract pathologist reinterpreted the materials of both a primary treating hospital and the district medical examiner. After finding a cogent cause of death, he then directly tested the parents, finding the relevant genetic evidence to support the anatomical finding of sickle cell disease (trait) in the decedent. A settlement for wrongful death followed directly. The intermediate connecting link in the pathogenetic scheme went unexplored: neither the primary hospital nor the medical examiner dissected the spinal cord at the site of anesthesia for evidence of possible direct intravascular injection of tetracaine hydrochloride, USP. Disinterment was considered but not attempted due to the rapid settlement.

Another case points to the usefulness of consultant pathologists in making confirmatory tests not undertaken during the initial study. A 55-year-old man had suffered for a number of years with refractory infections of the skin of the outer ear and of the auditory canal. These had been reasonably controlled by chloramphenicol, but other antibiotics as a rule were singularly unsuccessful. On the day of his death, he went without an appointment to see his regular physician, explained that while he had been on a trip the condition had flared up, and that a physician there had prescribed different antibiotics, to be taken topically and systemically. His regular physician, after some discussion on the toxicities of the drug, did prescribe chloramphenicol once again. Early that evening, while consuming an alcoholic beverage with friends in his kitchen, he stated that he had a pill (chloramphenicol) "caught in his throat," and then collapsed. He was attended within 15 minutes by an internist, who observed an open airway, a weak pulse that was profoundly bradycardiac, and deep cyanosis. Resuscitation was attempted, to no avail, and the body was removed to a nearby hospital foro postmortem examination. Prior to it, the body was embalmed by the bilateral supraclavicular technique (the "two point" system).

The past history of the patient included a possible heart attack at age 52. He was also known to have labile systolic hypertension. During the two-year period before his possible heart attack, he had twice been admitted to the hospital. The first time it was for an apparent allergic attack to chloramphenicol and certain grain foods to which he was also known to be allergic. The second time occurred after a meal that included tomatoes but no grain foods. This episode included urticaria, profuse perspiration, and pressing substernal pain that radiated to the jaw and both wrists from a point that was dorsal and mid-scapular. Both SGOT and LDH were elevated; and his systolic pressure peaked at 180 Torr. The symptoms were relieved by intramuscular meperidine and bed rest. One year before death his ear problem was relieved by the use of drainage tubes. The post-mortem examination confirmed an older myocardial infarction of the posterior papillary muscle of the mitral valve that extended widely across the posteroinferior part of the left ventricle. The heart was enlarged for body mass (500 grams); there was 50 percent occlusion at the bifurcation of the left coronary artery; 2 cm distal in the circumflex artery was another point of 50 percent occlusion of the inferior branch and 100 percent occlusion of a smaller, superior branch. The anterior descending and right coronary arteries were streaked but not narrowed. The gross lesion of greatest interest was narrowing of the larynx to 0.3 cm due to apparent extreme edema of the vocal cords and other parts of the mucous membranes of the hypopharynx. There was some mild pulmonary edema. The original investigation found eosinophilic leukocytes in the larynx, in the spleen, lung, and a few points elsewhere. The attending physician, cognizant of the probable past history of myocardial infarction and the labile hypertension, certified death as due to myocardial infarction and coronary artery disease. After the postmortem finding of swelling of the hypopharynx and vocal cords, this physician changed his death certificate to indicate death due to anaphylaxis. Detailed retaking of the immediate pre-ictal medical history indicated that the deceased had indeed taken one capsule very shortly before death; the exact time sequence could not be reconstructed. No sign of medications was found in the upper gastrointestinal tract at autopsy. Variation in stain intensity of myocardium was commented upon by the original pathologist.

The matter became a legal issue with the filing of a double indemnity claim on the basis of anaphylaxis related to chloramphenicol. The author was retained by the defendant insurance company, which did not agree to such payment merely upon filing. The case was tried in district federal court, with a resulting verdict for the company. The most pertinent evidence developed by secondary study was that the variability of myocardial staining was in fact a very striking fuchsinophilia by the Poley technique[24]. Interestingly, some few central nervous system neurones appeared acidophilic on hematoxylin and eosin and very strongly fuchsinophilic by the Poley method. It was opined on testimony that the swelling was the direct result of lower cervical embalming on a man with lax tissues, a change commonly observed by the author during training at Duke University, at which time embalming was a coordinated part of autopsy method. The eosinophilia was clearly a marker for long-standing allergic phenomena, but could not be invoked as evidence for a specific terminal event.

In this case, then, the contract pathologist performed additional tests that confirmed the leading cause of death, based on the general findings of autopsy and the details of clinical history, and ruled out as postmortem artifact a change invoked by some as the lethal lesion. In this case, another private consulting pathologist with extensive medical examiner experience agreed with the essential conclusions of the author and so testified.

A third case may illustrate the important value of detail as well as of familiarity with latent effects of traumatic injury, based on reinterpretation of autopsy findings. This will be mentioned only briefly here, since the full details of the case have been published elsewhere[28]. A 31-year-old man was involved as the "passive" victim of a rear-end automobile collision. His symptoms at first seemed related only to upper and mid-dorsal back and cervical strain, for which he was treated by the usual means, pain relief, collar support, and anti-inflammatory medications. Four weeks after the incident he was admitted to the hopsital *in extremis* with fulminant heart failure and hypothermia and died. Autopsy revealed anasarca and mildly increased heart weight. There was gross evidence for pulmonary edema. Upon reinterpretation, the myocardium revealed extensive intrafascicular edema and many small partially healed muscle fractures. The case was thus considered to be one of delayed cardiac contusion effects. CPK and

LDH were markedly elevated, and there were chemical signs of borderline renal dysfunction in the absence of specific lesions, points in favor of heart failure as the underlying cause of the problem. These points were elucidated during testimony in an action against the owner of the impacting car for wrongful death, an action which resulted in a verdict for the family of the decedent. In this case, no further tests were done by the contract pathologist. Rather, there was a fuller examination of the materials, competently gathered by the autopsy surgeon and interpreted from the perspective of broader forensic experience.

These three cases demonstrate the process of autopsy reinterpretation. It has been the common experience of the author that many hospital pathologists, whose appointments involve occasional medicolegal autopsy work, are reluctant to become involved in the actual legal process. No doubt many are reluctant because of time constraints, but some may do so because of sensitivity to local pressures. This was certainly true in the second case noted above. The original pathologist was most co-operative with the author (we knew each other in other professional contexts as well), but after the special studies cast doubt on the laryngeal lesion as significant, he was willing to testify only by deposition and was absent from the city during trial. The technical error was allowing pre-autopsy total body embalming. His autopsy procedure was otherwise done in a detailed and competent manner and provided the essential evidence for lack of recent ingestion of medication.

The five aforementioned cases represent a number of different ways in which private or nonaffiliated pathologists may serve in consultation to issues of legal importance. The final case in this section treated on the single issue of whether death was due to accidental or natural means. The contact to the author was from a life insurance company, which wished further elucidation pending a double indemnity payout.

Performance of Autopsy Following Disinterment

In 1958, a 51-year-old woman apparently fell and was supposedly unconscious for about 45 minutes. She had swelling of the left forehead and conspicuous black eyes for many days thereafter. X-ray found no fracture; the discharge diagnosis was severe concussion. After the incident, however, upon sudden physical changes in her position, she experienced blackouts lasting several minutes. Left eye vision began to fail and a diagnosis of traumatic neuritis of the first division of the fifth cranial nerve was established. Supraorbital neurectomy appeared to relieve the condition. At age 53, she was tested for possible brain tumor but no conclusion was reached. Eighteen months later, she apparently nearly drowned in a fresh water lake. Medical diagnoses in her general record included asthma and angina pectoris; the latter was sometimes relieved by nitroglycerine. On occasion of the near drowning, a great deal of water was inhaled and froth was present on her face and in her mouth when she was rescued and resuscitated. Brief hospitalization revealed no lung disease, and she was sent home. Almost exactly a year later she was sunning herself on a floating dock in a nearby lake; she was next observed to be in the water, motionless. Neighbors pulled her out but resuscitation was unsuccessful. The physician in charge remarked that he could not obtain water from the air passages. Nevertheless, a coroner's inquest concluded that she had in fact drowned, and burial was permitted.

The processing of the insurance claim was held up by the insurance company in question; they were dubious about the conclusion reached at the inquest. The author was contacted and agreed to perform an autopsy following disinterment. The body was identified by the funeral director, who was one of several witnesses. The externum was consistent with burial of three-month's duration in Florida soil. The body had been embalmed by both femoral ("one point") perfusion and much trocar injection. Despite the external decomposition, the internal viscera were well preserved, making histological studies possible, even including the brain, which was much shrunken. There was neither gross nor microscopic evidence for heart disease of the ordinary sort, and there was no pulmonary evidence for drowning. In fact, in the trachea the cilia were intact, extremely strong evidence against fresh water drowning. The thyroid was nodular with areas of hyperplasia, suggestive of possible past attacks of hyperthyroidism, which may have been interpreted clinically and by the patient as angina or asthma. The meninges revealed old blood pigment compatible with the remote trauma. This set of findings was interpreted to mean that she probably had an attack of tachycardia followed by asystole and rolled passively into the water from which she was rescued. On the strength of this report, the insurance company paid only the base amount of the deceased's policy, and her family did not pursue the matter further. In this case, the contract pathologist performed the primary autopsy, albeit after disinterment, and established the probable cause of death.

ACTING AS FORENSIC CONSULTANT TO CRIMINAL DEFENSE ATTORNEYS

This type of case uniformly came from attorneys in private practice after primary investigation, charging, and indictment but before trial. In some instances, the author's review of material took him to the office of the district medical examiner to study microscopical slides, and in one instance to examine retained gross tissues.

Apparent Drug-Releated Homicide

The author was brought into this case by a forensic psychologist working with a well-known criminal defense attorney, but many months after the alleged events. An emergency squad was called early one morning to a motel at an interstate highway interchange to assess a man apparently shut tight in a bathroom and making no sounds. The alarm had been raised by his girl friend when she had awaken. There had been some kind of drug use, probably including cocaine, the previous evening. The squad had to force the door, since the body was partially leaning up against it and, because the door, as is common in such places, only opened inward. When they reached him, the man's body temperature was in excess of 41°C, and he was not resuscible. The remains were turned over to the district medical examiner. The deceased was well known to the local drug circuit, and some evidence was uncovered that he bought cocaine the evening before. It was his habit to go to a motel, take the cocaine intravenously, strip naked, and then turn the shower on hot, running around the room with the gathering steam, polishing the furniture, or whatever. The woman confirmed that he had started in on these activities the night before. Various burns were found along his left wrist and forearm, over the left hip, and about the left ankle. Drug implements were floating in the bathtub, which contained tepid water to a depth of several inches. This evidence was given by an emergency technician who fell into the tub while attempting to assess the man's life status. Numerous photographs were taken of the scene and external aspects of the body. The burns were attributed to scalding, and the rectal temperature to cocaine kindling effect, since the amount of the drug actually in his blood stream was at the lowest level of sensitivity of the test method used.

The left-arm burns involved a coarsely oval area with bleb formation and peeling of epidermis. They suggested to me electrical burns rather than scald marks; there was no splash pattern. Nevertheless, the person from whom the man had apparently purchased the cocaine was located and charged with third-degree murder as well as sale of a controlled substance. When I visited the office of the medical examiner, I found no sections had been taken of the skin lesions. Blocks of the heart, however, showed segmental smudging of the fibers, which is seen sometimes in death by electrocution. At this point, I asked to be shown the scene of death. The room in question had been cleaned up, repaired, and painted because the right foot of the deceased, who had been found facedown, had punched a hole in the plaster board behind the bathroom door. We verified, however, that otherwise the basic configuration of the room had not been changed. As is often found in such buildings, the commode and tub-shower were in a small terminal room with one door, and the wash bowl or bowls were in an alcove leading to the toilet; this area had a wall mirror and shaver outlet, which in this case faced the sink but was on the same side as the alcove and toilet. The door jambs were steel, and the door strike plate fit perfectly with the pentagonal outline burn on the left hip.

It was immediately obvious to me what had occurred. In the victim's naked frenzy, cocaine induced or not, his skin had become damp from the steam in the shower. While he stood against the left side of the door jamb, his left wrist brushed against the duplex electrical outlet. The moisture in the air provided the contact and the arc exited from hip to strike plate and from ankle to broken paint near the floor, where shoes and mops had scratched the jamb. The photographs allowed measurement of the arm length and thus the precise location of the entry burn. This distance fit well with the location of the outlet a few inches above the countertop surface when a person was positioned at the jamb.

Based upon this interpretation given in deposition, the state attorney dropped the charge of murder against the defendant and entered a finding of accidental death by electrocution. The accused was given a year of supervised probation for the sale of cocaine. It was never determined, however, whether in fact the decedent had actually used the cocaine purchased the evening before from the defendant.

In this case, the consulting pathologist reinterpreted the autopsy findings by studying them closely *and* by visiting the scene of the death. The physical structure of the room and of the bathroom alcove and tub area in particular were conclusive with respect to a proper understanding of the findings. In fact, the fit of the burns was so precise in respect to the physical attributes of the room that I have since wondered how they could have been overlooked. It should be pointed out that the medical examiner had only examined the body and the police investigative team had only examined the scene of death with superficial attention to the burns. Somehow, the basic principle of dermatopathology seems to apply to such a case: the sections are often interpretable only by seeing the patient. This is a good maxim for death investigation generally, and essential for the after-the-event consultant. He or she is of course much dependent upon good photographic documentation during the primary investigation, and at least a modicum of detail in the autopsy report. In this case, no sections were taken of the burns; I prefer to believe that had such been done, the same conclusion would have been reached much sooner, and quite possibly without my involvement in the case.

Apparent Homicide by Shooting

Direct, personal investigation at the scene of an incident is vital for the forensic pathologist. It usually places him or her in a far better position to understand the interrelationship between medical findings and physical evidence. Sometimes, the scene is not intact and must be recreated, as for example when a motor vehicle is part of the incident. The case in question involved a shooting incident in which rather wide variations in blood alcohol determinations confounded the evidence. The gunshot wounds of the decedent were partially modified by emergency surgical efforts, and the accused assailant also sustained physical injury that required assessment for possible confirmation of his version of events. On the evening of the incident, three men went to a restaurant and bar on the outskirts of town. They arrived in a small truck and called themselves to the attention of the bouncer by parking askew two parking spaces. The latter asked them to put the truck in straight, and the driver did so. Perhaps 45 minutes later, the decedent made a public scene with his shirt and coveralls on the stage, and he and his companions were advised by the bouncer that they must behave or be arrested. After this event, the bouncer armed himself with a small handgun (.22 calibre pistol), putting it in his hip pocket. The three men got up to go, without actually being asked to do so. As they were leaving, one of them attempted to take a glass with a drink outside, and the bouncer asked him for it. The decedent threw it out of the doorway, and it broke on the pavement. As the bouncer came out, one of the other men threw a second drink at him, wetting his face and shirt. The driver was already in the truck, but a struggle began between the other two men and the bouncer. According to the bouncer, the decedent beat him, and he tried to break off the fight by using Mace, but was unsuccessful. The two men then dragged the bouncer farther out onto the lot, alongside the passenger side of the truck, at which point he drew his gun. The smaller of the two men retreated somewhat, but the larger man continued the struggle. The bouncer fired one shot. The struggle still kept up, but the bouncer was able to fire the gun twice more. The victim then staggered away about six feet and fell on his back near the rear of the truck. The second man then jumped the bouncer again, but the latter broke free, ran inside, and called the police. The victim was pronounced dead one hour later in a nearby emergency room, after a triaging transverse thoracotomy incision on the anterior left chest that cut across an apparent entry wound. The accused was also examined and found to have multiple contusions of a fresh nature on his back, with excoriations over the left shoulder, tenderness over the lower right ribs, and some irregular lacerations of the scalp which went deep to the galea. He was treated and then released into police custody.

The decedent was later examined at autopsy by the district medical examiner, and four gunshot wounds were found, but two were from the same bullet. They were numbered arbitrarily. Wound track #1 was described as a "contact range" perforating wound of the neck, with entry on the left anterior aspect just below the angle of the jaw. This was 0.25 inches in diameter, with abraded margins and a slight suggestion of muzzle imprint on adjacent skin. No residue of close-range gunfire was found, but abundant soot and flattened powder grains were present in the internal track, which went to the right through the strap muscles and base of tongue to exit just below the right angle of the jaw, perhaps slightly higher and rather more lateral than at entrance. Would track #2 entered slightly to the right of the anterior midline. This had a 0.75 inch circular soot and powder mark on the skin surface and was described as a close-range to loose contact wound. The track went backwards, slightly down, mildly to the right, and partially exited just beyond the crest of the shoulder on the dorsal side. The small calibre projectile was recovered from this site. The transit wound consisted of soft tissue injury and a narrow hemorrhagic zone about the track. Wound track #3 was a surgically marked left anterior thoracic injury 4.25 inches from the midline. Exploration at autopsy revealed an elongate guttering wound of the left ventricle that exposed the chamber, perforation of the apex, contusions of the left lung, perforation of the aorta, a posterior perforation of the right lower lobe, and massive hemorrhage in both pleural spaces. This bullet was found in the subpleural tissue of the posterior right thorax.

One account of the matter had the accused assailant simply firing his weapon;

unresolved was the possible alternate view that the decedent had jumped from the truck. It was clear that the wound track described as #3 was a disabling wound and was sequentially third. Actually *five* injuries were noted externally, since track #2 partially exited the skin. At all events, the various data provided the consultant with sufficient evidence to go forward with a scene recreation. The powder patterns ruled out shooting at a distance and at least partially confirmed the story of the accused; although the fatal wound entrance could not be satisfactorily studied forensically following surgical exploration, the other two could be, and the only satisfactory explanation of their greatly differing points of entry and passage was that they were incurred during intimate grappling by the accused and the victim. Inspection of the surface of the parking lot confirmed the nature of probable origin of some of the injuries of the accused, and his contusions the remainder. In his deposition the medical examiner stated: Q: "Would you expect that wound to cease any fighting or resistance on the part of a victim in a struggle?" A: "Not necessarily. I would anticipate a person having received that wound would still be able to maintain a fight or flight activity for a short period of time." Q: "Up to what range?" A: "Less than a minute." In other words, a disabling injury. The confusion over the blood alcohol arose when the primary state laboratory reported a urine level of 180 mg/dl and a blood level of 240 mg/dl. A reference laboratory at some distance reported 400 mg/dl; just prior to his deposition ten months after the incident, the state laboratory chemist repeated his test on a stored sample and found 380 mg/dl. These are differences too large to account for fully by simple variations. The prosecution originally claimed the higher reference figure would make the victim incapable of such a struggle, but the overall results and the closer coordination between urine and the first state lab result from blood surely meant they were more likely accurate; the time interval of visitation to the bar would support the belief that renal equilibration had not yet been achieved. After thorough discussion of all these points, the attorney for the accused obtained dismissal of the homicide charges, and a plea of *nolo contendere* to aggravated assault was entered.

Here the consultant forensic pathologist was a reference source for the attorney for the defendant, providing technical information on trajectory analysis, alcohol testing, and the injuries of the accused to help produce a coherent view of what happened. The medical examiner was unwilling rather than unable to draw a conclusion as to how the injuries were sustained. For his part, defense counsel was content to obtain confirmation of descriptive detail, relying on the consultant to reconstruct the most probable course of events. His reconstruction sufficiently confirmed the story of the accused that the above-noted result occurred. Of particular value was experiential literature on the technical problems with postmortem blood or tissue alcohol determinations[3,15].

Apparent Child Abuse with Death

At a critical moment in *The Hound of the Baskervilles*, Stapleton and Holmes have just met on the moor over the body of Seldon, the escaped convict. Stapleton presses Holmes for an explanation of the puzzling occurrences, but Holmes replies: "One cannot always have the success for which one hopes. . . . It has not been a satisfactory case"[13].

Likewise, even diligent and thorough investigation by a forensic consultant may not lead to a satisfactory resolution of a case. In this one, the problem lay not with the consultant but rather with the emotional and psychological torment of persons who felt they had been wrongfully accused. The couple in question were middle-class individuals with a successful business and sufficient community standing to be granted provisional adoptive custody of three children. These were natural siblings who had been put up together for adoption through a state agency by their natural mother to protect them from the stresses of separation, a working mother, and a reportedly alcoholic father. The adopting mother was a former teacher with good letters of recommendation. The decedent was a five-year-old boy with siblings six and seven. The boy was brought to an emergency room in haste, with the adoptive father driving and the adoptive mother giving mouth-to-mouth resuscitation in the face of obvious vomitus. The boy died several days later with clinical evidence of intracranial bleeding. Cutaneous contusions evolved over the hospital course and numerous photographs documented the details. Erythema of the perineum was observed but not of the lateral or gluteal areas.

It was revealed that the adoptive parents had used to discipline the child by having him sit exposed in a sink of water of uncertain heat. No specific dermal evidence of this having occurred recently was found, however, despite the mother's story that the boy had taken a bath by himself and appeared to have been scalded and then bruised while attempting to get out of the tub. He had been found facedown in the bathtub the previous evening, but was easily aroused by the mother—who got there first after hearing his screams (she was near the kitchen door)—and since he didn't seem in distress was not taken to hospital until the next morning, when he awoke and began vomiting.

In deposition, the medical examiner said he could not imagine the extent of injury as being due to a fall in a bathtub, even if there had been thrashing around in a vigorous way. The author was called into consultation. The two adoptive parents were charged at different times; the other children were removed from their home and put elsewhere. The adoptive father, absent from the house at the time of the bathtub incident, was arrested seven months after the events. Local headlines were large. After a preliminary study of the police reports, the autopsy record, some evidentiary depositions, and the statements of the accused, the author visited the house and spent several hours talking with the parents and examining the bathtub. Numerous measurements, diagrams, and photographs were taken from inside the tub, from the bathroom into the tub, and through the window for other angles. A doll model of the boy was made to standard dimensions, and on a second visit of several hours was tested in the site for further study. The timing of the mother's response was recreated, at great emotional toll.

The microscopical sections from the autopsy were examined in detail, and I then met with the medical examiner in the presence of the prosecutor and the parent's respective private attorneys. Several additional factors were presented and the retained organs not previously examined were jointly studied by the examiner and the author. Several added blocks were submitted. The most significant of these were of the epiglottis. These revealed resolving inflammatory lesions of a type and character strongly suggestive of acute obstructing epiglottitis of an age, considering the duration of maintenance by respirator, fully compatible with the interval in question. From the numerous and generally excellent photographs, it was possible to reconstruct a map of contusions. Every one of them could be accounted for by the specific characteristics of a bathtub—the soap dish, the spigots, faucet, drain, inside towel bar on the sliding glass door, etc. Internal lesions could also be explained by comparable points in analysis.

Despite the wealth of detail these investigations produced, there was continued legal maneuvering. Over a year after my personal investigations were completed, and more than three years after the incident, the couple failed to appear for a formal hearing on possible changes in charges, and have not been heard from, or of, since. It is clear that they had reached their breaking point. One of the two defense attorneys provided me with this update when I asked after the disposition of the case. There was a interval of sixteen months between my final report and the inquiry.

The details in the case are numerous and cannot be provided here. When the medical examiner said he could not imagine how the injuries could have been inflicted by the boy himself, he did so without recourse to having done what I did later: stand and squat in the tub itself, Polaroid(R) camera in hand, working with tape measure, rulers, pad, and pencil. His report, however, was detailed and valuable. The inner extent of certain contusions, when compared to their surface character, gave some further insight into the probable angle of impact. Between us, we provided a complete investigation, one which perspective suggests should have been made in the first place. Again, the forensic pathologist is in a superior position, with the requisite knowledge of the tissue lesions, to understand how things occurred, but only if the site is examined critically.

ACTING AS FORENSIC CONSULTANT TO PUBLIC DEFENDERS

In this capacity, the consultant pathologist does all of the same things noted in the previous section, but, because of the nature of the systems involved, is often called upon very late in the judicial process.

Apparent Homicide

This case bears more resemblance to the one described earlier concerning the shooting in the parking lot, insofar as the autopsy evidence required critical interpretation, than it does to the case of electrocution, which involved misapprehension of cause. A woman was found dead in her front yard, savagely struck about the face and head, but with food in her stomach and 50 ml urine in the bladder. The food contained partially digested vegetables. She was found midmorning by a neighbor. Evidence developed that another neighbor had had soup with the decedent just before 7 P.M., watched television, and went home at 7:55 P.M. The body was quite cold when found facedown. Her stepson had mowed the lawn that afternoon. He lived elsewhere with a girl friend, a point of contention with the decedent. He arrived on the scene during the height of the police investigation, became hysterical, and could not account for an apparent blood stain on the floor mat of his girl friend's car. He said he had visited his mother between 10 P.M. and midnight, had found her well, and that she had been alive when he left her. At first, the medical examiner, who visited the death scene as part of the police investigation, opined that death occurred very shortly after the meal in question. He later placed death as occurring at around 11 P.M., the interval during which the stepson said he was with the deceased.

After being charged with the death of his stepmother, the man changed his story. He was a convicted felon, an accessory in an incident during which a policeman had died, and he had served some time in jail. He now said that he came back to his stepmother's house at the time he previously said she was all right, found her dead on the front lawn, coming very close to the body to make that determination himself, panicked, and fled the scene. He surmised that the would be charged with her death even though it was known they had a good relationship.

The woman's two natural children knew him, were supportive, and believed in his innocence. The critical issue then became how reliable was the evidence on time of death. The accused had a good and supportable alibi up to 10 P.M., but by his own admission was on the premises sometime during the final two hours of the day. Jewelry was missing, but could not be traced to him. There was no question about the lethal wounds, only their timing. Based on the neighbor's testimony about the specific character of the meal, and the stomach and bladder findings, the author's opinion was that death was very close in time to the neighbor's departure. Others in the neighborhood had returned home around 10 P.M. and heard nothing going on at that time. It seemed reasonable enough that the fluid load of the soup had not yet promoted an accumulation of urine. On repeat deposition, the medical examiner offered some collateral findings from rigor mortis and algor mortis, but these points were not very precise.

It was developed that the second opinion was after the stepson had been taken into custody. At the time of trial, after the prosecution had rested, the public defender represented to the judge on motion for directed verdict what the consultant's testimony would be: confirmation of the medical examiner's initial opinion, the interval for which the accused had a supportable alibi. There were also some other problems in the evidence not of a medical nature, and the motion was granted and not appealed. The consultant did not actually testify.

That homicide had been done was unmistakable. What could not be shown by the evidence available was that the stepson, a convicted felon, had committed this crime. His conduct was seen as reflecting his understandable fear of being charged; in his panic he was either unaware of his footprint containing the victim's blood on the floor mat or he chose to let the incriminating evidence remain. The latter is rather incomprehensible behavior for a man of his experience with the criminal justice system; it would seem rather that he found her body sometime after the murder, and late in the evening at that, so that he was unaware of his getting blood on the sole of one shoe.

In this case, the forensic consultant served to reinterpret data in evidence on the death interval[17,25,26,33].

Apparent Child Neglect

A functionally illiterate school janitor and his deaf mute wife had two natural children, a boy about eighteen months old and an older girl. The girl was thriving and seemed to show no learning problems, considering the family circumstances. The boy, though, was not thriving physically. A home health visitor advised the parents to take him to the county health clinic, but they did not do this, and he fell gravely ill and died. Autopsy revealed an obvious marasmus, which was somehow interpreted as due to their withholding food from the child, the evidence of the sister notwithstanding. Autopsy photographs and microscopial slides were sent to the author. These revealed, among other things, a great deal of hemosiderin in the liver, spleen, marrow, and in some other connective tissues. A primary disorder causing hemolytic anemia could not be discerned from the meager medical history. Some of the features of the case suggested the Zellweger syndrome[23] and others a transferrin deficit or anomaly. There seemed to be sufficient evidence of death from natural causes to result in the dropping of manslaughter charges that had been filed. Because the parents had failed to affirmatively respond to the instruction from the health visitor, a year of supervised probation was ordered on a charge of child neglect. It is unclear to the author just how a visit to a county clinic would have reversed an untreatable genetic disorder.

In this case the principal role of the consultant was interpretation of the evidence and, in particular, the autopsy findings.

Apparent Manslaughter in an Automobile Incident

A young adult woman, previously married, had an argument with her current boy friend that was overheard at least to externals by fellow patrons at a restaurant bar. Threats were reported to have been made. The couple then left the scene, and the only further particulars of the story come from the accused. He stated that she mauled him and spilled beer on him while he was trying to take her home. Her purse was thrown from the car. (It was later found.) He stopped the car once; she threatened to jump out, a threat she had also once made to her former husband, who was living in a state far distant at the time of the incident. The accused decided to take her to a hospital, concerned that a possible head injury from a fall some weeks before might somehow still be affecting her. He admitted to slapping her to try to calm her down, but she only doused him with beer again. Then, as he drove toward the hospital at an estimated 50 miles per hour, she jumped out. At the time, they were driving along a typical Florida highway with sandy grass shoulders. After she jumped, he was able to stop and turn the car around. He drove back to the scene, found her well over on the grassy shoulder on her back and, despite the blood on her face and in her mouth, he began to give her mouth-to-mouth breathing. Alternately, he tried to flag down another car. This took a long time, as was later reconstructed comparing the times given in his own account with those of the people who had overheard the argument at the restaurant.

A rescue squad physician pronounced the girl dead at the scene, and autopsy was done in due course. Numerous photographs of the marks and injuries on the body were taken, most of them of some evidentiary value. The medical examiner found intracranial blood, hemorrhage about the cervical cord (as viewed through the foramen magnum only), a laxity of the upper cervical vertebrae, and symmetrical bilateral tears of the cerebral peduncles.

After reviewing the evidence, including the photographs, the author attempted to discuss the case with the medical examiner, but he refused, and subsequent questions were transmitted through the public defender. On the morning of trial, I was able to closely inspect the automobile, which had been impounded, and turned out to have belonged to the decedent.

Evidence technicians had gone over it before, and their report was available. The decedent was a motorcycle devotee and had been weaaring a homemade necklace of hard metal that included washers and hexagonal nuts. A rolling injury was present on her neck that corresponded well with this piece of "jewelry." She had hard impact contusions on her left side at the flange of the pelvis and to a lesser extent on the forearm. The left boot was scuffed sharply along the outer side. Her right mandible was fractured with minimal surface contusion, and the superior ramus of the right hyoid bone was fractured inward. No comparable lesion was found on the left. There was ecchymosis of both orbits and a number of other surface marks; the metallic buttons of her jacket had fresh, sharp scratches.

The defendant was charged with severely beating her, in specific fracturing her jaw and right hyoid bones, and thereby causing her death. The official report did not describe four significant marks on the car: (1) a sharply etched loss of paint on the inside trailing edge of the jamb near the upper limit, a mark with a particular pattern very crudely shaped like an "F" and fitting the dimension of the necklace; (2) a dent on the metallic ledge of the passenger window (this was a 1974 Vega) that was the same distance from the flared lock button (3 inches approximately) as the distance from the mandibular fracture to the hyoid fracture; (3) an impact mark on the anterosuperior edge of the rear wheel housing (the fender is raised less than an inch) that was the same distance from the possible necklace mark as was the neck wounds related to the necklace were from the hip impact contusion; and (4) an impact wiping of grease from the lower inside edge of the passenger door with sharp indentations that conformed to blue jeans the victim was wearing that had grease on the right side (i.e., possible seam impacts). I later took photographs of the marks and changes on the car; at the time I inspected it in the custody lot, the right door was locked. It seemed reasonably clear that as she went out the door, attempting to put her feet out so as not to jump on her head, the relatively great weight of the door plus the wind force against it caused her head to be caught in the upper corner, breaking her neck and tearing the cord (this could not be checked out as the cervical cord was not dissected at autopsy). Her left side then slapped hard against the car, scuffing her boot and bruising her hip. The accused must have slowed the car down at this point, with the door opening slightly from its own momentum. This caused her head to slide down against the closed glass window (several pictures showed a soft compression bruise with fairly sharp edges on the forehead) and with great force she struck her chin and hyoid bone more or less simultaneously on the appurtenances of the door. She then dropped ventrally onto the pavement and from momentum rolled directly onto the grassy shoulder, coming to rest on her back. Blood ran down onto the collar of the jacket and onto the upper shoulder arc as well.

The injuries were interpreted by the prosecutor as evidence of her head being banged by the accused, even though there was no scalp contusion at that point. The changes in the peduncles were undoubtedly postmortem artifacts from hasty removal of the brain, a change the author has seen more often than he cares to remember, especially when trainees have go at it; no microscopic studies were made to identify the character of the edges of these tears. The jury was not shown the marks on the car, leaving the photographic evidence unbalanced.

Despite a Florida appellate holding that the accused's account of events has to stand in the absence of any other witness to the incident, the jury found him guilty. In this case, subject to possible retrial or appeal, the consultant's efforts have served to clarify the means of dying, but not necessarily a full determination of the instrumentality of death. In my opinion, the lethal injury is well explained by this hypothesis of occurrence; the relative forces are akin to excessive twisting of forceps on the fetal head, leading to transection of the cervical spinal cord[29].

As a consultant long after the fact, I could study the body only from reports and photographs. Some of the latter were excellent. The injuries were clearly more severe than those from a direct fall out of an automobile, given the known character of the roadside. Inspection of the car, something the medical examiner had not done, produced findings not recorded by evidence technicians and accordingly not part of the early official attempts to investigate the case.

However, four months after trial, the court, citing the above mentioned Florida apellate holding and the details of the evidence herein described, dismissed the conviction for manslaughter while leaving intact the conviction for aggravated assault, which is on appeal.

Thus I come full circle, seemingly critical of the performance of official medical examiners in a wide variety of cases. Since the majority of forensic autopsies are done by hospital-based pathologists whose training is predominately on adult cases, the matters involving children may seem to warrant earlier consultation—before charges are filed. I know of such cases and the procedure is to be commended. In many instances, however, the actual data gathering by the medical examiners has been good and in fact vital to later reconstruction of the case by the consultant. The appearance of confrontation is to a reasonable degree the presently inescapable result of the too-close affiliation between the offices of medical examiners, both full-time and part-time, and the prosecutorial arm of the judiciary. This is both a public perception and a practical reality. Greater support for and genuine independence of the investigative function are both much needed. Whether a supplemental, national corps or agency would help is unproven for lack of same, but it *would* strengthen the independence factor. Establishment laws could be drawn more precisely. In Florida, the counties must underwrite their own activity; this probably should be a state system set up on a district base, more like that now found in Tennessee, but with direct state support. University affiliation would not only enhance the exposure of other health care trainees (and law students as well) to the field of forensic sciences, but would provide access to other disciplines of occasional pertinence to forensic investigation. Such agencies would be affiliates of the universities, and the examiners would hold academic rank in those parts of the system actually on or near the campuses.

Failing the above, the increased activity of private consulting forensic pathologists and other forensic specialists may serve to assist in creating improvements in the field, especially those directed toward enhancing the involvement of the pathologists in the detection of information outside of the autopsy room and away from the laboratory. Forensic pathologists can be the integrative factor in better investigation. It is just as wrong to falsely accuse as it is to overlook a case, whether civil or criminal, in which culpability can be established. We owe our best efforts to society at large, lest it become one in which "the dead must bury their dead" without even scriptural metaphor[32].

In this article, from the personal experiences of the author a variety of situations representative of those in which a private consulting forensic pathologist might become involved has been illustrated. Such cases are always challenging, hardly ever dull, and characteristically offer one some unusual opportunities for new insight, the kind that one might, in fact, expect, from one's position as an unofficial personage.

REFERENCES

1. Ahronheim, J. H., "How it works: the medical examiner system." *Michigan Medicine*, May 1977, 271–73.

2. Bennett, R. C., "The changing role of the coroner." *Canad. Med. Assoc. J.* 118:1133–38, 1978.

3. Blackmore, D. J., "Ethanol and aircraft accidents," *in* Mason, J. K. and Reals, W. J., *Aerospace pathology*, 1973, Coll. Amer. Path. Found., Chicago, Chapt. 21, pp. 203–210 (*vide*, especially pp. 206–207).

4. Connelly, R., *Dr. John D. Rogers v. the Medical Association of Georgia, the Composite State Board of Medical Examiners, and Governor George D. Busbee*—an update. *J. Med. Assoc. Georgia 68*:997–98, 1979.

5. Corrigan, G. E., Realm of forensic pathology (letter). *N. Eng. J. Med.* 279:48, 1968.

6. Curran, W. J., "Medical-examiner system in Massachusetts." *N. Eng. J. Med.* 282:556–57, 1970.

7. Curran, W. J., "The status of forensic pathology in the United States." *N. Eng. J. Med.* 283:1033–34, 1970.

8. Curran, W. J., "Medicolegal investigational systems: new demands of the 1970s." *N. Eng. J. Med.* 284:30–31, 1971.

9. Curran, W. J., "Ethical and legal problems in medical participation in criminal investigations." *N. Eng. J. Med.* 294:764–65, 1976.

10. Curran, W. J., "Forensic medical science: the continued problems of judges and juries." *N. Eng. J. Med.* 294:1042–43, 1976.

11. Curran, W. J., "Damage suits against medical examiners for authorized autopsies." *N. Eng. J. Med.* 197:1220–21, 1977.

12. Doyle, Sir Arthur Conan, *A Study in Scarlet*, in *The Complete Sherlock Holmes* (standard reference edition), 1953, Doubleday & Co., New York, Vol. I, p. 17.

13. Doyle, Sir Arthur Conan, *The Hound of the Baskervilles, Ibid*, Vol. II, p. 875.

14. "The dying detective." An unsigned editorial in *N. Eng. J. Med.* 278:1176, 1968.

15. Francisco, J. T., and Baldwin, T. E., "Are postmortem alcohols valid?" *Medical Times* 100:145–55, 1972.

16. Helpern, M., "Fatalities from child abuse and neglect: responsibility of the medical examiner and coroner." *Pediatric Annals* 5:42–57, 1976.

17. James, W. R. L. and Knight, B. M., "Errors in estimating time since death." *Med. Sci. Law* 5:111–16, 1965.

18. Jason, D., "Broadening of existing medicolegal office legislation." *Legal Med. 1980*:137–148, 1980.

19. Lippsitt, P. D., "Medical inquiry and the law." *N. Eng. J. Med.* 277:974–75, 1967.

20. Luke, J. L., Requirements of Forensic Pathology(letter). *N. Eng. J. Med.* 278:1178, 1968.

21. Luke, J. L., "Forensic pathology." *N. Eng. J. Med.* 295:32–34, 1976.

22. Opinion, Illinois Attorney General, "Duties and powers of the coroner's office." *Ill. J. Med.* 155:19, 1979.

23. Opitz, J. M., et al., "The Zellweger syndrome(Cerebro-hepato-renal syndrome)." *Birth Defects* 5:144–60, 1969.

24. Poley, R. W., Fobes, C. D., and Hall, M. J., "Fuchsinophilia in early myocardial infarction." *Arch. Pathol.* 77:325–29, 1964.

25. Rose, E. F., "Factors influencing gastric emptying." *J. Forensic Sci.* 24:200–206, 1979.

26. de Saram, G. S. W., "Estimation of the time of death by medical criteria." *J. Foren. Med.* 4:47–57, 1957.

27. Shanklin, D. R., "The master's methods in medical detection; five case studies

of the utilization of observation and deduction in the realm of forensic medicine.'' *Grimpen Mire Gazette* 1:10–14, 1981.

28. Shanklin, D. R., ''Delayed fatal impact cardiopathy.'' *Foren. Sci. Internat.* 25:283–91, 1984.

29. Shulman, S. T., Madden, J. D., Esterly, J. R. and Shanklin, D. R., ''Transection of the spinal cord. A rare obstetrical complication of cephalic delivery.'' *Arch. Dis. Childh.* 46:291–94, 1971.

30. Sopher, I. M., ''The medical examiner system: a new concept in community medicine for the State of West Virginia.'' *West Vir. Med. J.* 72:49–55, 1976.

31. Taylor, B., ''The case of the outspoken medical examiner.'' *Maryland Med. J.* March 1977, 59–69.

32. *The Bible, Mat*, 8, 22 and *Luke*, 9, 60.

33. Van Den Oever, R., ''A review of the literature as to the present possibilities and limitations in estimating the time of death.'' *Med. Sci. Law* 16:269–76, 1976.

34. Wecht, C. H., Realm of forensic pathology(letter). *N. Eng. J. Med.* 279:48, 1968.

35. Wecht, C. H., Forensic pathology—a specialty in trouble. An editorial in *N. Eng. J. Med.* 297:1232–33, 1977.

2. Homicide Investigation—Importance of Scene Visit by Forensic Pathologist

Cyril H. Wecht, M.D., J.D.

In May 1981, at the end of the spring semester at Carnegie-Mellon University, Dr. Wen-chen Chen, an assistant professor in the Department of Statistics, his wife, Su-jen, and their one-year-old son, Eric, returned to Taiwan to visit their families. Dr. Chen was planning to return to the university in early July to carry out his summer research program. However, on Friday, July 3, word was received that Dr. Chen had been found dead early that morning on the campus of the National Taiwan University in Taipei. He had reportedly been interrogated at length the previous day at the headquarters of the Taiwan Garrison Command, the powerful security agency of Taiwan's ruling party, the Kuomintang.

The initial press reports that reached the United States quoted officials at the Garrison Headquarters as stating that Dr. Chen probably committed suicide by jumping from the fifth floor of the fire escape of the graduate school research library at National Taiwan University because of his antigovernment activities and "because he feared being arrested for his crimes." These officials claimed that Chen admitted creating ten foundations in the United States to raise money for *Formosa* magazine, a dissident journal published in Taiwan that had later been shut down for alleged sedition. These reports immediately generated strong reactions of disbelief and suspicion at Carnegie-Mellon University and elsewhere throughout the United States. The mysterious circumstances surrounding Dr. Chen's death continue to be the subject of speculation by the worldwide news media.[1]

The death of Dr. Chen exposed the political strains existing among the Taiwanese at home and abroad. Major factors that have led to the current unrest include the resentment of the native Taiwanese at mainland domination of the political system and the resistance of intellectuals to the tight security controls imposed by the government to prevent Communist subversion and antigovernment activities. Although these strains are due in part to the economic and political difficulties that all modern societies face, the recent history of Taiwan has been such that the character of its present political tensions is somewhat unique.

The population of Taiwan has been almost completely Chinese since the twelfth century. Japanese domination of the island following the Sino-Japanese War in 1895 had little effect on the Chinese traditions of Taiwanese society, and was brought to an end in 1945 when the Chinese regained control. Taiwan was then ruled by the Chinese Nationalist Government of Chiang Kai-Shek and became the seat of the government after the Communist takeover in 1949 forced the Chinese Nationalist mainlanders to seek refuge in Taiwan.

Although in the minority then and now, the mainlanders have continued to reserve to themselves the controlling positions in the government, the Kuomintang party, and the military.[2] This dominance was originally justified in terms of the stated national objective, mainland recovery; it has been perpetuated by an official policy which holds that, since the government represents all of China, it should not be dominated by the Taiwanese. Many Taiwanese, however, view this policy as a mainlander device to retain power, and have responded with demands for independence. Although advocates of independence have been unable to create effective underground organizations in Taiwan, several Taiwanese independence organizations were formed abroad over the years, with chapters in many countries, including the United States, and with memberships composed primarily of Taiwanese students.

Taiwan has been under martial law since 1949, and as part of its internal security program, the government has prohibited as subversive all organizations favoring Taiwanese independence. Furthermore, any questioning of the political system or the mainland recovery policy by the news media is forbidden, and several political periodicals published in Taiwan and judged to be subversive by the Kuomintang have been suspended, shut down completely, or forced to change management. The Taiwan Garrison Command maintains an extensive network of informants and watches for any suspicious activities or evidence of disloyalty. There have been recent allegations that the Garrison Command also uses its surveillance network to monitor the activities of the 500,000 Taiwan citizens currently residing in the United States.[3]

In light of the ever-present Communist threat to Taiwan, most citizens support the use of security measures; however, there is also some fear that these may be carried to excessive lengths, resulting in the lack of legal protection for the ordinary citizen. To date, the mix of "repression and reform" has stayed within the limits acceptable to the majority of people in Taiwan but, as noted by Ralph Clough in his study of Taiwanese politics:

> Many would like to see a more representative national government, greater freedom for public debate, and a relaxation of security measures. Some of those pressing for change

are among the American-educated intellectuals who have returned to Taiwan from the United States in increasing numbers during the past few years.[4]

The mainstream of the Taiwanese Independent Movement overseas now emphasizes the need for democratic reform, rather than the overthrow of the Kuomintang and the Nationalist Government. Internally, however, there continues to be little government tolerance for the independence movement. Thus, although the Taiwanese living in the United States who have contributed to the support of the Taiwan-based *Formosa* magazine may have done so in the hope of bringing about reform, government authorities nevertheless linked the magazine to the Taiwan Independence Movement, convicted its founders of sedition, and sentenced its general manager to life imprisonment.[5]

Dr. Chen, who was outspoken in his support of a more democratic Taiwan while a student and professor in the United States, found himself in a perilous position when he returned to Taiwan on a family visit. He was interrogated there by the Garrison Command, not as a proponent of reform, but rather as an anti-Kuomintang activist. The question of whether his death a few hours after his questioning was an accident, a suicide, or a politically-motivated homicide remains unanswered. In an effort to learn moroe about the circumstances surrounding the death of Wen-chen Chen, Professor Morris DeGroot, Chen's colleague in the Carnegie-Mellon Statistics Department, and Cyril H. Wecht, M.D., J.D., a forensic pathologist and former Allegheny County Coroner, travelled to Taiwan in September 1981 to examine the scene of the death and the body of Dr. Chen.

The trip was prompted initially by a telephone call in late July to Dr. DeGroot from a fellow professor of Statistics in the United States with contacts in Taiwan. This call conveyed the request of several interested and concerned members of Taiwan's governmental and academic circles that DeGroot visit Taiwan in order to obtain a better understanding of the facts relating to Chen's death. Chen's widow, who had returned to Pittsburgh with their son, Eric, in August, informed Dr. DeGroot that Chen's father and other family members also felt a trip to Taiwan would be helpful. Several members of the United States Congress, both in the House of Representatives and the Senate, as well as various officials of the State Department, shared this opinion and encouraged a trip if the government of Taiwan would give its permission.

The trip was discussed, and arrangements were completed by September 16. The Taiwanese government agreed that Dr. Wecht could accompany Dr. DeGroot and that he would be permitted to carry out an examination of Dr. Chen's body. It was also agreed that both men would be allowed to meet with government officials, family members, and others connected with the case. A telegram confirming the visit was received from Taipei the following day and, after being supplied with visas, DeGroot and Wecht left Pittsburgh, arriving in Taipei on the evening of September 21.

During the three-day visit, DeGroot and Wecht met with Dr. Chen's friends and family; several Taiwanese professors; the director and staff members of the American Institute, which serves as the unofficial United States Embassy in Taiwan; various government officials, notably Yun-suan Sun, the premier of the Republic of China; and General Ching-hsu Wang, the head of the Taiwan Garrison Command. It must be emphasized that during all these meetings, as well as throughout their entire stay in Taiwan, DeGroot and Wecht were received with the utmost in courtesy, hospitality, and genuine concern. A great deal of information was obtained from these meetings, as well as from the various examinations that followed, all conducted with the permission of the Taiwanese government.

Dr. Wecht had the opportunity to perform a second autopsy on Chen and, while at the Taipei coroner's office, where the original autopsy had been performed on July 6th, he also was permitted to examine Chen's gross organs. The microscopic tissue slides prepared from the original autopsy and the results of toxicological tests were made available to him for examination as well as at the laboratory of the investigation bureau of the Ministry of Justice. During the course of their visit, DeGroot and Wecht also made a careful and detailed inspection of the site where Chen's body was found. Thanks to the cooperation of Chen's father, an examination of the clothing worn by Chen at his death was also made possible.

Throughout his stay in Taiwan, Dr. Wecht was accompanied by Director Chou of the Foreign Affairs Division of the Taipei police, who provided security and personal protection with ability, graciousness, and consideration. Three Taiwanese professors served as his hosts and guides: Dr. Kao-wen Mao, the president of National Tsing Hua University, who received his Ph.D. from CMU in 1969; Dr. Chun-shan Shen, a professor at National Tsing Hua University; and Dr. John M. Fong, a forensic pathologist at National Taiwan University College of Medicine. Dr. Fong trained for a year in forensic pathology and legal medicine at Harvard University in the mid–1960s, and had been in telephone contact with Dr. Wecht prior to the trip. Dr. Wecht believes that these three professors offered their help and cooperation, not as representatives of their government, but as individuals who wished to express their concern for the tragic death of another academician whom they held in high respect. It appeared that they genuinely believed that the Taiwan government was not officially involved in Chen's death, and they were anxious to demonstrate this to Dr. Wecht.

The information obtained as a result of conversations with Chen's family and friends and meetings with government officials primarily addressed the two issues central to this case that have yet to be resolved: were Dr. Chen's activities in the United States and Taiwan seditious, and what precisely was the manner or legal cause of his death?

There seems to be a consensus as to the events of the day preceding Chen's death. On July 2, Chen, his wife, and child were staying at the third-floor apartment of his brother-in-law, waiting for the required exit visas to be processed so they could return to the United States. At approximately 8:30 A.M., representatives of the Garrison Command arrived at the residence and requested a voluntary interview with Chen to discuss alleged involvement with the Taiwan Independence Movement in the United States. This requested interview is referred to by the Garrison Command as a "yueh tan," literally, an "appointment to talk" requiring the person's permission. Refusal is, theoretically, possible. However, Chen agreed to be interviewed, and at 9:00 A.M. he arrived at the Command Headquarters. The interview continued until 9:30 P.M., when Dr. Chen was escorted back to his brother-in-law's by a special Command vehicle. Although the escort walked him to the second floor of the building, Chen never arrived at his brother-in-law's apartment. Taiwan officials claim that he apparently waited for the special vehicle to leave, and then walked a short distance to the home of Wei-hsiang Teng, an associate professor at the National Taiwan Institute of Technology who, together with his wife, Grace, were friends of the Chen family. Teng has stated that Chen did not arrive at his home until 11:00 P.M. or later, leaving some mystery as to what occurred between approximately 10:00 P.M. and 11:00 P.M. Once at Teng's, Chen ate a small meal and briefly discussed the events of the day with his friend. Teng remembers Chen writing a letter and having it in his hand when he left Teng's home; the letter has never been seen or received in the mail, as far as anyone knows.

Six hours later, at 6:30 A.M. on July 3, Chen's body was discovered outside of the graduate school research library of the National Taiwan University. There remains a great deal of contention over what occurred in the course of Chen's interrogation at the Garrison Command, where or with whom he spent time after leaving Professor Teng's home, and how and when he actually died.

Although the government says that Chen fell or jumped from the fifth floor fire escape of the library, on the evening of Dr. Wecht's arrival in Taipei, Chen's father and brother-in-law met with him and emphasized their dissatisfaction with this explanation and with the investigation of the case by the authorities. The following evening, Dr. Wecht met with Dr. Jam-erh Pai, a professor of Business Administration at Taiwan University, and a friend of the Chens. Su-jen Chen had called him early in the morning of July 3, indicating that her husband had still not come home and asking for his help. His attempts to ascertain the whereabouts of Chen resulted in contradictory answers as to when Chen had been released by the Garrison Command. He was first told that Chen had been released at about 9:00 A.M. that morning, July 3, but later, through other channels, he learned that Chen had been released at about 9:00 P.M. on July 2. Pai stated at this meeting that he was sure Chen had no reason to commit suicide.

Immediately after the conversation with Pai, Dr. Wecht met with Dr. Teng and his wife. Teng reiterated his recollection of what occurred during Chen's visit to his home the night of July 2, and emphasized that Chen showed no indication of contemplating suicide. Furthermore, he is of the opinion that Chen would have had no reason to go to the top of the fire escape of the library, either to think things over or to meet someone.

There are obviously widely disparate opinions as to the manner of Chen's death. The same situation exists regarding the question of whether Chen was involved in seditious activities, either abroad or in Taiwan. Colleagues of Chen from Carnegie-Mellon University have stated that he was not active in any anti-Kuomintang movement in the United States. In confirmation of these opinions, no evidence that Chen did anything of a seditious nature in regard to the Taiwan government was presented to DeGroot and Wecht while they were in Taiwan. Nothing was elicited or volunteered during the course of the entire investigation that would suggest, and certainly nothing that would prove, with even a modicum of evidence, that Chen was involved in any kind of treasonous activities, or even activities that might be considered harmful to the government.

The government apparently disagreed, since the subject of their 12½-hour-long interview with Chen was his alleged involvement in the *Formosa* magazine sedition case that had earned the defendants sentences from 12 years to life.

Dr. Wecht obtained a great deal of information on this issue in an extended meeting with General Wang, the commander of the Taiwan Garrison General Headquarters, and Colonel Chou, chief of the Investigation Section of the Garrison Command Security Department, and the officer who had carried out the interrogation of Chen. These individuals were extremely cooperative, and Dr. Wecht's 5½-hour meeting with them was quite productive.

During the meeting, Dr. Wecht listened to a 15 or 20 minute-tape recording that covered the last part of the Chen interrogation. He also reviewed a written transcript of this recording, and was later given a 12-page handwritten transcript, which he was told summarized the important parts of the interrogation. Chen's signature was on each page of the transcript.

General Wang and Colonel Chou responded to questions posted by Dr. Wecht and made the following points:

I. The Taiwan Garrison General Headquarters wanted to interrogate Dr. Chen because their investigation of the Kaohsiung incident (a riot that occurred in December 1979, allegedly instigated by the Taiwanese Independence Movement) showed that he had been involved in fundraising activities for *Formosa* magazine.

II. They waited until shortly before he was ready to return to the United States before calling him in for interrogation because they did not know until he visited the Exit and Re-entry Processing Administration (ERPA) on June 30 that he wanted to leave Taiwan in early July. Until then, they had assumed that Dr. Chen, like most other professors visiting Taiwan during the summer, would not want to return to the United States until late August, and they did not want to bother him during his visit with his family.

III. Dr. Chen's interrogation on July 2 was, in fact, his first interrogation at the Garrison Headquarters. The ERPA, where he had been questioned on June 30, is under the auspices of the Department of the Interior, whereas the Garrison Command is run by the Department of Defense.

IV. The four main points established during the interrogation of July 2 at the Garrison Headquarters were as follows:

1. Dr. Chen stated that he helped set up foundations to raise money for *Formosa* magazine.
2. Dr. Chen stated that he transmitted funds that were collected to Shih Ming-teh, the General Manager of *Formosa* magazine.
3. Dr. Chen stated that, in Pittsburgh, he helped to arrange for the translation into English of an article in *Formosa* magazine.
4. Dr. Chen stated that during his visit to Taiwan, he had spoken to various people about the question of establishing democratic reforms. Of these four points, the Garrison Command regarded the last one as the most serious because they were concerned that Dr. Chen had returned to Taiwan to express antigovernment sentiments.

V. The Garrison Command was not planning on filing any charges against Dr. Chen when they released him and sent him home following the interrogation. They had indicated to him that they would try to facilitate his departure for the United States.

VI. The Garrison Command does not have any letters that Dr. Chen sent to Shih Ming-teh, nor do they have any other documentation showing that Dr. Chen sent money to Shih. They do not have any recordings of speeches or comments that Dr. Chen made in the United States. They do have a recording of a telephone conversation between Dr. Chen in the United States and Shih in Taiwan, because Shih was under investigation for criminal activities, and his telephone was monitored.

VII. The Garrison Command did not put much pressure on Dr. Chen during this interrogation, and he was in a pleasant mood when he left the Garrison Headquarters.

VIII. Dr. Chen was not kept under surveillance, either before or after his interrogation by the Garrison Command.

IX. The Garrison Command does not know where Dr. Chen was between the time that they released him at approximately 9:30 P.M., and the time that he reportedly arrived at the home of Dr. Wei-hsiang Teng at approximately 11:00 P.M., or where he went when he reportedly left Dr. Teng's home at approximately midnight.

X. Chen did not ask to be allowed to make a telephone call to his family during the interrogation, although in accordance with Garrison Command procedures he would have been permitted to do so.

XI. The district attorney of Taipei refused to meet with Dr. Wecht and Dr. DeGroot during the visit to Taiwan because the case is still officially open, and he is in charge of the investigation. To act otherwise could disturb the legal status of that investigation.

It should be emphasized that there is no indepedent way of verifying the accuracy of these responses. For example, the exact relationship between the ERPA and the Taiwan Garrison Command is unclear. From the questioning of Chen on June 30 and July 2, and the fact that three agents of the Garrison Command picked him up on the morning of July 2, when he had been told to expect a call from the ERPA, it would appear that the two organizations are in close communication with each other.

The question of whether Chen was involved in any activity which could be construed to be seditious by government officials is, of course, important when considering whether Chen's death was an accident, suicide, or homicide. This is particularly true in view of the many allegations by political groups and family friends that Chen was murdered as a result of his dissident behavior. As noted above, there has been little concrete evidence unearthed to substantiate the government's position that Chen died by accident or by suicide. For example, no one that DeGroot and Wecht spoke to, including family, friends, and high government officials, when asked in a friendly but firm, probing fashion, could point to anything that would have laid the psychological groundwork for this man to have taken his life. Furthermore, it has never been satisfactorily explained why newspapers quoted Garrison Command spokesmen immediately following Chen's death as saying that Chen had probably committed suicide for his crimes and that they had evidence of these "crimes." For both Wang and Chou told DeGroot and Wecht that no crimes had been committed by Chen and no evidence of crimes existed.

The final analysis and ultimate conclusions, however, must be based, as much as possible, upon the physical evidence, the scene inspection, and the examination and physical findings of the body. Putting all these things together, a forensic pathologist can evaluate an unnatural death, consider the three possible manners of death—accident, suicide, and homicide—and then try in a logical fashion to arrive at what is the most likely answer. Fortunately, during his stay in Taiwan, Dr. Wecht had the opportunity to make important preliminary examinations before coming to his conclusions regarding the manner and circumstances of Chen's death.

THE AUTOPSY

On the evening of his arrival in Taiwan, after a 24-hour trip from Pittsburgh, Dr. Wecht was conducted to the Taipei City Funeral Parlor by Chen's father; Martin Tai, Chen's brother-in-law; an escort from the American Institute staff; and Dr. Shen and Dr. Fong. There, starting at midnight, a thorough, detailed, and complete examination of Chen's body was made. The body had been kept frozen, and there was no significant deterioration in its condition from that observed in photographs taken during the autopsy performed on July 6 by Dr. Fong and two other government physicians. Dr. Fong is a forensic pathologist who had acted as a consultant to the government for this particular autopsy; the other two doctors were in fact police surgeons.

Both the outside and the inside of the body were fully examined. Incisions that had been made during the July 6 autopsy were reopened, and new incisions were made where it was felt that supplementary information could be obtained. In particular, the midline of the back was dissected from the cervical to the coccygeal region. Throughout the examination, Dr. Wecht asked Mr. Chen and Mr. Tai to point out any injuries about which they were particularly concerned, and special care was taken to investigate these injuries.

The following comments were made by Dr. Wecht during the autopsy:

Dried ice covers the head, face, and neck completely, as well as much of the upper anterior chest, arms, forearms, and hands. The ice is removed by prying, gentle tapping with forceps, and application of warm dripping water. The body is photographed in situ with the ice present, and then rephotographed after almost all the ice has been removed. Various photographs of the body were taken during the autopsy.

Multiple postmortem incisions from the original autopsy are noted over various portions of the body. These include the following areas:

1. Right lateral neck area extending from the lobe of the right ear downward and slightly anteriorly, ending in the right supraclavicular area.
2. An incision over the medial-lateral aspect of the right clavicle.
3. A lengthy incision from the midline of the chin down the anterior midline of the body, ending in the pubic escutcheon.
4. An incision on the lateral aspect of the right elbow which is V-shaped. One branch continues laterally and posteriorly above the right elbow while the other continues laterally, dorsally, and downward below the elbow joint onto the upper dorsal aspect of the right forearm.
5. An incision on the antero-lateral aspect of the right knee.
6. A lengthy incision extending from the upper left lateral aspect of the symphysis pubis down along the anteromedial aspect of the left thigh, ending at the medial aspect of the lower left thigh at the suprapatellar level.

The midline of the back is dissected from the cervical to the coccygeal region, revealing extensive hemorrhage in the dorsal and lateral paravertebral musculature beginning in the lower thoracic vertebral area and extending downward into the sacral region. Liquid blood is present in this area, diffusely distributed throughout the subcutaneous tissue, musculature, fascial and ligamentous structures.

Palpation of the spinous processes reveals definite mobility at approximately the L3 level, indicating a fracture.

It is not possible to remove the vertebral column because no saw or other appropriate instruments are present. However, in light of the extensive hemorrhage and fracture of the spinous process of the third lumbar vertebra, it is quite conceivable that the spinal cord would have been contused, and possibly even lacerated to some extent.

The somewhat linear abrasions of the right side of the back, which are diagonally oriented, with the lower margin being located toward the posterior axillary line and upper margins more toward the midvertebral line, show hemorrhage into the underlying subcutaneous tissue upon dissection through the epidermal abrasions.

In the region of the right upper flank, the hemorrhage is much more extensive and diffuse, extending into the underlying musculature as well as the adipose tissue. There is not continuous hemorrhage from the right upper flank area to the lumbar vertebral area of hemorrhage. Some underlying subcutaneous tissue and musculature were spared for the most part from the traumatic injuries that produced these extensive areas of hemorrhage and the fracture of the third lumbar vertebral spinous process.

The face is carefully examined, and there are no injuries of any kind. The conjuctivae are clear. The auditory, nasal and oral cavities show no obstructions. The lips are carefully examined and no abrasions or lacerations are seen. The teeth are in a good state of repair and show no loosening, hemorrhage of the gums, or other injury.

There is hemorrhage in the mid-to-lateral supraclavicular region noted in the subcutaneous tissue and musculature. This hemorrhage is essentially subjacent to an area of contusion hemorrhage noted on the skin surface in the right lateral clavicular region.

There is a small amount of hemorrhage near the symphysis pubis and a fracture with minimal separation of the pubic bones at their juncture.

The wrist, hands and fingers are carefully examined and no specific injuries are seen except foor a few superficial abrasions on the anterolateral aspect of the left lower forearm approximately two to three inches above the left carpal level. Dissection through these areas shows only minimal hemorrhage into the underlying subcutaneous tissue and focal extension of hemorrhage into the musculature beneath.

The fingernails are intact and show no loosening. There is dark, uniform bluish-purple to bluish-black discoloration of all the fingernail beds, consistent with postmortem cyanosis. Exaggeration of this color change is secondary to dehydration and postmortem decomposition.

No defensive injuries of any kind are seen on the hands and fingers.

The feet and toes are carefully examined. The toenails are intact, and dull reddish-purple to purplish-black discoloration is noted, although not quite as dark as the color seen in the fingernail beds.

The upper and lower extremities show no gross deformities, nor is there any crepitus or abnormal movement noted on passive motion of the extremities.

The fingernail of the left forefinger is removed by carefully dissecting the lateral margins and the proximal base. The nail is then pried loose from the underlying subungual soft tissue. The area shows dull reddish-brown discoloration consistent with postmortem change and some postmortem cyanosis. The area is smooth with no apparent abrasions, lacerations, or focal hemorrhage. The undersurface of the nail is then examined and found to be smooth and intact with no evidence of fractures or tears. No antemortem hemorrhages are seen on the inner surface of the nail.

The rib cage is examined. The right fourth rib is fractured in the anterior midclavicular line. The right fourth, fifth, sixth, and seventh ribs are fractured in the anterior axillary line with some displacement. The seventh, eighth, and ninth ribs on the right side appear to be fractured in the posterior line approximately three inches to the right of the costovertebral junction. Associated hemorrhage is seen in the intercostal musculature in conjunction with these various rib fractures, most noticeable posteriorly.

The cervical vertebrae and thoracic vertebrae show no evidence of fractures, although there does appear to be some hemorrhage in the intercostal musculature extending to the costovertebral junctions at the T4 to T7 levels.

The antecubital fossae of both arms are carefully examined, and there is no evidence of recent or old needle marks. An incision is made into the antecubital fossae, and no hemorrhages or old track marks are seen in the underlying subcutaneous tissue.

A fairly transverse fracture of the undersurface of the sternum is noted in the midline at the level of the fifth rib. The fracture extends from one side to the other across the midline, but does not go further across the sternochondral junctions. Additionally, there is a fracture of the lower left portion of the sternum involving the sternochondral junctions of the left seventh, eighth, and ninth ribs. Definite mobility is seen in this area when the sternum is held firmly in one hand and manipulated with the other.

The anteromedial aspect of the left thigh is dissected and laid open from the femoral region to the suprapatellar level, and no hemorrhages are noted in the underlying musculature.

A dissection is made of the medial inferior margin of the anterior surface of the right knee, representing the site of the abrasion-contusion seen on a previous photograph and described in that area. No deep hemorrhage is present in the underlying musculature.

The viewing of the body was concluded at 2:15 A.M.

Later in the trip, Dr. Wecht visited the Taiwanese Minister of Justice Bureau of Investigation. This is an excellent new facility located at the distant southern end of the city. He was greeted by the director of the Laboratory Section, the deputy director and some department chiefs, including a young man who was a graduate of the FBI Academy in the United States. This was the facility where the toxicological analyses were done on Chen's blood. The facility is extremely well-equipped, and the top-level personnel appeared to be intelligent, well-trained, and familiar with postmortem toxicologic analyses.

The toxicological studies that had been done were negative. The very small amount of alcohol in the blood found in these analyses was most probably due to some postmortem decomposition changes. The 0.4 mg percent level of alcohol is insignificant and irrelevant scientifically, though perhaps it might be found to relate to where Chen might have been, and with whom, and when he might have eaten, etc. (Dr. Wecht, however, believes it was most likely a postmortem artifact.) Although these toxicologic studies, to the extent they were conducted, were negative, the examiners could have tested for some other compounds. Unfortunately, that was not done, and Dr. Wecht was not permitted to take tissues back to the United States for testing.

At this same facility, forty-five microscopic autopsy tissue slides from Chen's postmortem examination were made available to Dr. Wecht. A fine Vickers microscope was present, and Dr. Wecht examined all the slides. The significant histological findings were as follows:

1. Diffuse pulmonary edema and pulmonary hemorrhage.
2. Focal areas of mononuclear inflammatory cells, principally lymphocytes, suggesting that death did not occur for at least twenty to thirty minutes. There is no cellular infiltrate into the alveolar spaces.
3. The remaining organs are unremarkable, except for some minimal fatty change of the liver.

A trip was then made to the central morgue facility in the city, where the coroner-medical examiner's autopsies are done. This was the facility where the original autopsy on Chen was performed by Dr. Fong and his two colleagues.

At this site, the gross organs were made available to Dr. Wecht. They were well preserved, wrapped in gauze, and placed in a large bucket filled with formalin. The following findings were reported by Dr. Wecht:

1. The right lung showed focal areas of hemorrhage and focal lacerations at the dorsolateral surface. The left lung showed minimal foci of hemorrhage.
2. Heart unremarkable.
3. Spleen unremarkable.
4. Liver unremarkable, except for a suggestion of slight fatty change.
5. Left kidney unremarkable; right kidney, several slightly jagged lacerations present on the dorsal surface in the mid-portion projecting in toward the hilum.
6. Urinary bladder unremarkable.
7. Brain and dura matter unremarkable.
8. Tongue, neck organs, including thyroid, portions of strap muscles, trachea and upper bronchi, all attached. Unremarkable.
9. Stomach unremarkable.
10. Gastrointestinal tract unremarkable.

EXAMINATION OF PHYSICAL EVIDENCE: CHEN'S CLOTHING

On the evening of his second day in Taiwan, Dr. Wecht met with Chen's father and brother-in-law to examine the clothing worn by Chen when he died. The six pieces of clothing had been kept in a large plastic bag and included Chen's jockey shorts, gym shorts, slacks, shirt, shoes, and belt. Each item was carefully inspected by Dr. Wecht, who made the following observations:

The white jockey shorts had been cut on both sides of the elastic waistband, presumably by the investigators who removed the clothing from Chen's body. There were also five defects that appear to have been caused by cutting with scissors. Presumably, these were areas that were removed because they contained noticeable or suggested stains.

The yellow gym shorts have a white nonelastic band and two white pull-strings protruding from holes with metal circular borders. There is a pocket on the right front with a white top that is not closed. A defect is seen in both the right front and right rear areas. Both appear to have been made with scissors.

A pair of light blue men's slacks with a very tiny checkered pattern has been previously cut down the mid-line back seam from the waist into the crotch. Numerous stains can be seen on various portions of the slacks in the buttocks area, both in the mid-line on the left and right, more so on the right. Various stains are present along the right lateral pants leg, the right knee area to a slight degree from the right upper medial thigh region near the crotch, on the left lateral lower thigh area, and over much of the left knee region.

A brown leather belt with a metallic buckle shows no defects.

The pair of white leather men's loafers with a metallic buckle on each, with the word "LUCK," are slightly scuffed and somewhat dirty, but otherwise unremarkable.

A pale blue, short-sleeved men's dress shirt (Arrow, 100 percent cotton, 15½ neck size) has buttons down the anterior mid-line and one pocket on the left upper front. The front of the shirt is unremarkable and the short sleeves are intact. The back of the shirt has some stains on the rear part of the left sleeve and some dirt marks on the back part of the right sleeve. Also present are some similar, rather light, diffusely spread stains in the upper part of the shirt on both the left and right sides of the mid-line and connecting through the mid-line portion.

Two somewhat linear, irregular stains on the right side of the shirt are grossly parallel to each other and appear to be separated by a distance of approximately six to seven inches. These marks and the distance that separates them are consistent with the abrasion-contusions noted on the right side of Chen's back, as depicted quite clearly in the photographs that had been sent previously to Dr. DeGroot, and in the photographs contained in a bound booklet, presumably prepared by Dr. Fong as part of the postmortem protocol, which had been viewed earlier by Dr. Wecht. The lower area of staining is associated with an extensive tear of the shirt that extends from the left side and moves slightly downward in a diagonal plane, ending at the right lateral seam of the shirt. According to Chen's brother-in-law, the tear is more extensive now than was originally noted; however, a tear was present in this area originally. Other diffuse, irregular staining can be seen in the lower part of the back of the shirt.

It is important to note that the right upper anterior shoulder portion of the shirt is essentially clean, with no demonstrable stains or scuff marks, although in this area some contusions and slight abrasions of the right mid- and lateral clavicular region were noted on the body.

INSPECTION OF THE SITE

Very early on the morning of his final day in Taiwan, Wecht, accompanied by Dr. Shen, was joined by Dr. Fong on the campus of the National Taiwan University for an inspection of the site where Chen's body had been found. This time of day was chosen because it would be light enough to see things easily, but too early for the campus to be crowded with students.

The cars were checked at the gate and, after identification, the party proceeded

Figure 2.1

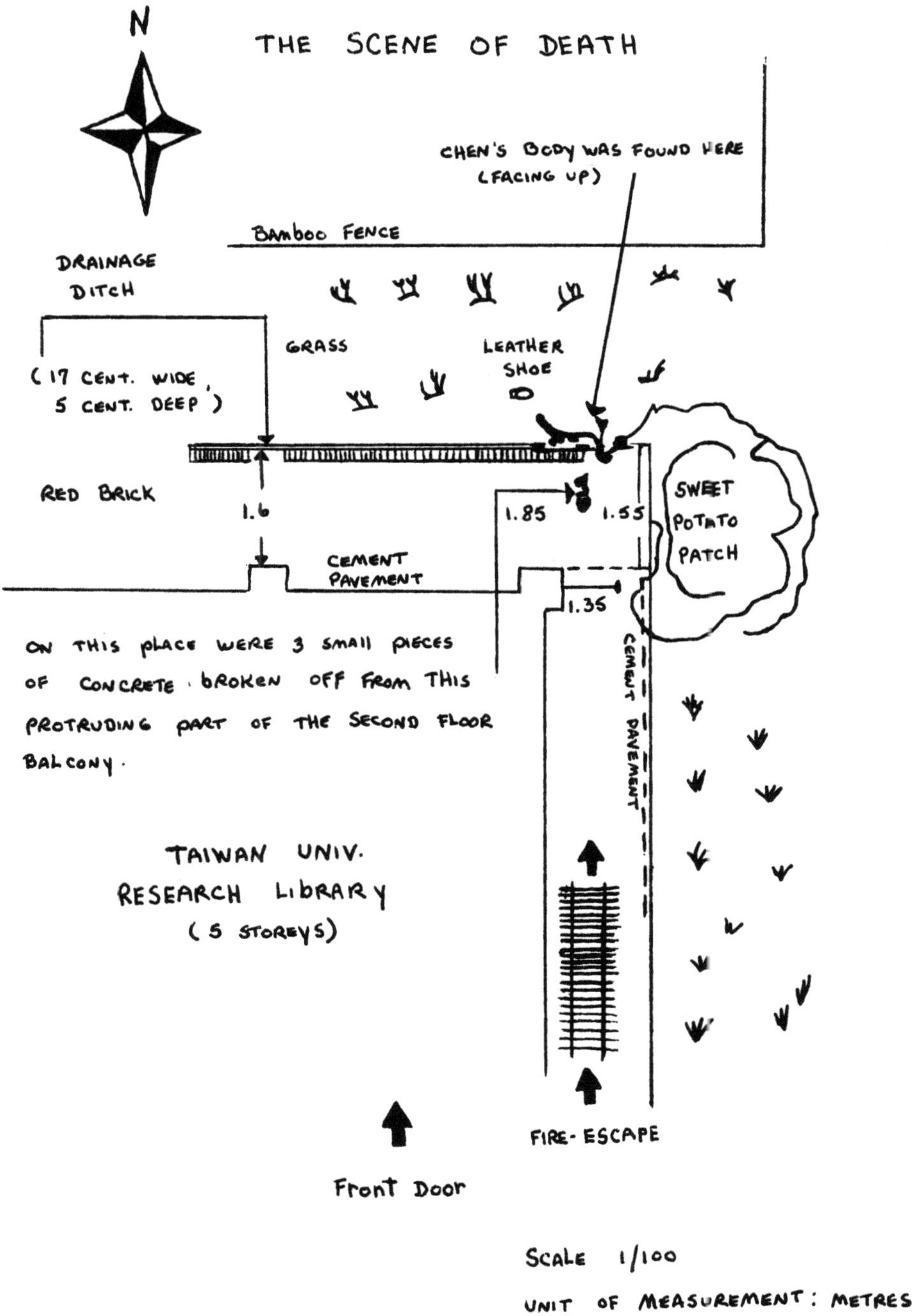
N
THE SCENE OF DEATH
CHEN'S BODY WAS FOUND HERE
(FACING UP)
BAMBOO FENCE
DRAINAGE
DITCH
GRASS
LEATHER
SHOE
(17 CENT. WIDE,
5 CENT. DEEP)
RED BRICK
1.6
1.85
1.55
SWEET
POTATO
PATCH
CEMENT
PAVEMENT
1.35
ON THIS PLACE WERE 3 SMALL PIECES
OF CONCRETE BROKEN OFF FROM THIS
PROTRUDING PART OF THE SECOND FLOOR
BALCONY.
CEMENT PAVEMENT
TAIWAN UNIV.
RESEARCH LIBRARY
(5 STOREYS)
FIRE-ESCAPE
Front Door
SCALE 1/100
UNIT OF MEASUREMENT: METRES

into the campus, arriving a few hundred meters away at the graduate school research library. The library is a five-storey, grey, concrete and white, brick building with an external stairwell at its northeast corner. At the northeastern corner of the building where the body was found, there is a shallow ditch, only seventeen centimeters wide, with a brick border on both sides. The red, elongated bricks, situated in a perpendicular fashion to the ditch, can be seen readily on the side proximal to the building. There are, however, some patches of grass and earth on the bricks at this side and, in fact, they partially cover some of the bricks in the area where Chen's body was found. The brick on the side farther away is completely covered over by grass and cannot be seen or felt unless the grass is parted. The ditch itself is approximately five centimeters deep. Although the grass was slightly moist that morning, no water was present in the ditch, in spite of the fact that there had been a substantial amount of rain for two days in Taipei.

Along the side of the ditch closer to the building, numerous irregularly shaped pieces of broken glass are present, as well as many small irregularly shaped stones and other pieces of debris. On the far side of the ditch, the ground has a slight upward tilt at an angle of perhaps five to ten degrees. There is a cement walkway at the northeast corner of the library that is 160 centimeters wide from the edge of the concrete pillar to the edge of the proximal row of bricks that line the ditch.

The fire escape or external stairwell begins along the eastern side of the building toward the northern end. The width of the stairwell is 26 inches (66 centimeters). The railing is iron on both sides, painted black, and the stairs are poured concrete. Although it is quite comfortable for one person, two people could not walk up these stairs abreast unless they were small children. On the first floor landing, the height of the railing is approximately 31½ inches (80 centimeters). The concrete landing protrudes 27 inches (69 centimeters) from the base of the iron railing. There are two chips at the outer rim of the concrete edge. These two defects are approximately 35 inches (89 centimeters) apart. There is a door on the second-floor landing and on the fourth-floor landing, but none on the third floor. There is a landing between the fourth and fifth floors with no door, and then a landing on the fifth floor with a door. The fifth-floor landing is approximately 90 inches (227 centimeters) in length along the eastern side and 34½ inches (88 centimeters) wide at the northernmost corner. The railing is 32½ inches (83 centimeters) to the highest point. (This is at the level of the upper thighs below the symphysis pubis for Dr. Wecht, who is somewhat taller than Chen.)

It should be notoed that all the railings have what appears to be fairly fresh black paint with no chipping or flaking. It is reported that the railing was painted after the incident on July 3.

Looking down from the fifth-floor landing to the area where the body was found, the second-floor landing protrudes two feet farther out in a northerly direction than the fifth-floor landing, and the concrete walkway and the grassy patch can be seen. A voluntary jump or leap from the fifth-floor landing would almost certainly have taken the body beyond the width of the concrete walk, causing it to land on the grass. A person stumbling over the railing accidentally would quite likely have cleared the concrete walk area, because of the momentum that the body would have if it fell over the railing. On the other hand, a body simply picked up and dropped from the fifth-floor landing would probably have landed on the concrete walk, for two reasons. First, it would be somewhat difficult for one person to hurl a body any farther away from the building. Secondly, an individual can easily see in broad daylight that the concrete walk is close to the building, and that the earth is grass covered from the other side of the narrow ditch. Therefore, if the appearance of suicide is desired, the body would be dropped onto the concrete rather than onto the grass. Or, assuming that an individual was not dead, but merely dazed or unconscious from whatever cause, and death was intended to occur as a result of the fall, then it would be evident that the body would have to be dropped onto the concrete in order to insure substantial traumatic injuries. Even a lay person could see that if the body were to fall onto the grass-covered earth, the injuries incurred might not be sufficient to produce death.

On July 1 and 2, there had been academic examinations for the students at the university. These terminated on the afternoon of the second. Thereafter, students were not on campus for any academic purposes. Faculty examiners grading the test papers on the morning of July 3 occupied a white brick building directly behind the north side of the library building, There were university police is the area, more or less to maintain the academic security of the examiners' building.

The graduate school research library building is readily accessible, one side fronting the main street of the campus. There are no fences or gates around it, except for a bamboo fence at its northern border that separates it from the white brick building in which the examiners were located on July 3. The base of the stairwell from the ground floor has no gate or any other hindrance that would impede an individual's entering the stairwell. However, the campus security enforces curfew rules after 11:30 P.M., since this is the dormitory restriction hour on campus for girls. There are no restriction hours for males. From 11:00 P.M. to 7:00 A.M., however, cars are not allowed to drive onto campus without special permission. This would imply that no car containing Chen, alive or dead, conscious or unconscious, could have driven onto campus. Records are kept at campus police headquarters for any vehicles that do not receive special permission to enter the campus between 11:00 P.M. and 7:00 A.M. These records show that no vehicle was permitted to enter the campus on the late night of July 2 or early morning of July 3. However, despite the official policy requiring records of vehicles entering the campus late at night, there is a possibility that if occupants of a car flashed their credentials at the guard at the gate, they might have been permitted to enter without question or written record of their visit.

After 4:00 A.M., daytime activities commence, with people coming to exercise, walk, etc., and no restrictions are enforced after that time of day. It should be noted that, at this time of the year, July 3, daylight begins around 4:00 A.M.

Jen-fu Liu, the campus police guard who had been sent by the campus police headquarters to investigate a report that a person had been found lying near the library, described the position of Chen's body when he found it at 7:20 A.M. on July 3. He indicated that the body was lying in a supine position across the ditch. The head was pointed in a northeasterly direction, away from the library building, so that the left arm and left leg were on the proximal side of the ditch, and the right side of the body was on the far side of the ditch. Liu stated that the left arm was flexed at the elbow away from the body with the hand facing down toward the lower left hip region. The right arm was stretched more or less straight out, with the hand a few inches from the body. The legs were spread somewhat apart and, as he remembers, the shoe was present on the left foot. He did not notice the right foot because it was hidden in the grass. After determining that the body was not that of a sick or drunk person, but rather of an apparently dead individual, he immediately went to call his superior officers. He did not move the body. The official investigators arrived at the site at 10:45 A.M., July 3 and, according to official reports, this was the first time that the body was moved from the position in which Mr. Liu found it. However, pictures taken at that time show that both elbows were flexed upward. According to Chen's family, the site was not properly cordoned off and made secure in anticipation of further investigation.

After meeting with Liu and inspecting the ground and fire escape, Dr. Fong, Dr. Shen, and Dr. Wecht travelled through the campus and noticed the freshman classroom building a short distance from the graduate school research library. It has a larger, wider external staircase that goes to the top of what appears to be a six-storey building that is at least fifty feet higher than the fifth-floor landing of the library. The entrances to this building and to the external stairwell are closed by a metal door that completely blocks any access after 9:30 P.M. However, the gate to the building is opened sometime in the early morning to let in the cleaning people. Once one is inside the building, the stairwell to the second floor enables one to go through a connecting walkway over to the external stairwell.

On both sides of the base of this external stairwell, there is a wide concrete or cement walkway. This site would, therefore, appear to be more appropriate than the graduate school research library for anyone contemplating suicide who had a personal knowledge of the campus buildings, as Professor Chen did.

CONCLUSIONS AND RECOMMENDATIONS

The report of the autopsy performed on Chen on July 6 is accurate. The qualifications of the individuals involved in the autopsy were generally impressive, the quality of the microscopic slides was good, the preservation of the organs and the body was good, and there was no indication of anyone at the professional level attempting to obfuscate the physical evidence in this case. Furthermore, the physical injuries, external and internal, that were found in Dr. Wecht's autopsy were essentially identical to those that had previously been visualized, commented upon, and listed as diagnoses in Dr. Fong's autopsy report. However, since that autopsy was not done until three days after the death, and because the scene had been disturbed and all of the physical evidence on and surrounding the body had not been evaluated by criminalistics experts, not as much was learned from the examination as was possible. At that time, Dr. Fong had not concluded that Chen's death was a suicide or an accident, but felt rather that death had occurred in an undetermined manner. Although Dr. Wecht certainly had to consider the possibility of accident or suicide, the examination of the scene and of all the physical evidence presented during the course of the trip provided an extensive scientific foundation upon which to base his conclusion that Chen's death was a homicide.

No evidence was found of systematic torture having been applied to Chen. In the examination carried out on the night of September 21, Chen's fingernails and toenails were found to be intact, and no injuries to the fingers or toes were found. Dark discoloration of the fingernail and toenail beds consistent with postmortem cyanosis was noted. One fingernail was removed by dissection, and it was noted that neither the nail nor the underlying tissue showed any injuries.

The contusions on the left forearm and the cluster of small puncturelike abrasions on the right elbow were carefully examined and found to be superficial. These abrasions are not believed to be needle marks. It was suggested by the Taiwanese pathologist, Dr. Fong, that these marks could have represented ant bites made while the body had lain on the ground prior to its discovery. However, it is more likely that these abrasions were caused by the fall. The area onto which the body was thrown is quite rough, and strewn with numerous pieces of glass, small rocks, and other debris. Anyone falling from a standing position, even a child running and playing, could be marked similarly. And a body that is hurtled through space to land on such a surface is more than likely to get such multiple abrasions. A body landing with that kind of force could even get abrasions from the tall shards of grass. There were tall, fairly firm blades of grass, at least a foot high, present at the site. Although the body would crush them, the blades of grass could produce abrasions on the body in a cluster if that part of the body were to land on such a surface.

A further dissection was made at the location of the contusion near the right-knee injury, and this contusion was also found to be superficial with no deep hemorrhage present in the underlying musculature. This contusion could have been caused when Chen's knee bumped against the railing when his assailants attempted to lift him over it. Finally, the width of the brick gutter across which Chen's body was lying when it was discovered on the morning of July 3 was found to be the same as the distance between the two parallel linear abrasions on his back.

The physical evidence and the injuries that have been observed indicate that

Chen died as a result of dropping to the ground from an upper floor of the fire escape of the library. An early antemortem cellular reaction observed in the microscopic tissue slides indicates that Chen was alive at the time of the fall and lived for at least 20 to 40 minutes after the fall. The time of death is uncertain, but can be inferred to have occurred between 3:00 A.M. and 6:00 A.M., based upon the absence of food in the stomach and the findings of rigor mortis and livor mortis made later that morning. This conclusion as to the timing of death, based on the absence of food in the stomach, is predicated on the acceptance of Teng's account of Chen's late night visit to his house.

There are three possible explanations of this unnatural death: suicide, accident, or homicide. As stated above, no one with whom Dr. Wecht talked in Taiwan believes that Chen committed suicide. The members of his family do not believe it, his friends do not believe it, and the officials of the Taiwan Garrison Command do not believe it. Wecht was repeatedly told that neither his general personality nor his mood and outlook on the night of July 2 were suicidal.

No plausible explanation of how the death could have been an accident has been presented. Students of National Taiwan University sometimes go to the top of the fire escape to cool off on a hot night or to be able to talk privately. However, the fire escape and cramped platform at the top are clearly visible from the steps of a nearby building. It does not seem that this platform would be a comfortable or private place to go, either to be alone or to meet someone else. There is no reason to believe that Chen would have gone there in the middle of the night for either of these purposes.

Furthermore, neither the location of the body nor the pattern of the injuries support the explanation of suicide or an accident. A suicidal leap from the fifth floor would very likely have carried the body farther away from the library building and farther out onto the grassy area than was observed. An accidental tumble from the fifth floor would also have carried the body farther out than was observed. Either a suicidal leap or an accidental fall would typically result in observable injuries to either the arms or legs that were not present on Chen.

On the other hand, both the location of the body and the pattern of injuries are consonant with the explanation that Chen's body was held in a horizontal position over the railing of the fire escape and dropped onto the ground below. One or more persons holding Chen in such a position and striving to cause serious injury or death would attempt to drop the body close to the building so that it would fall onto the cement walkway or brick gutter nearby, rather than onto the grassy area farther away.

It is possible that Chen's body struck the edge of the protruding platform on the second floor of the fire escape as it fell. It is stated in the Taiwan's prosecutor's report that three cement flakes found on the ground near the body match the defects on the chipped edge of the platform. During the inspection of the site, the authors noted that the second-floor platform does protrude beyond the platforms of the higher floors, and that several indentations were present in the chipped edge of the second-floor platform, some of which appeared relatively new and others relatively old. It is more likely that this platform would be struck if Chen were dropped close to the library building than if there were a suicidal leap or an accidental fall.

The fact that there were no signs of a struggle and no signs that Chen twisted or tumbled or shouted during his fall, and the fact that he lived for approximately 20 to 40 minutes after the fall, all lead to the conclusion that he was probably unconscious or dazed when he was dropped. He was a strong man, and this was a limited space. It would have been very difficult for his body to have been dropped if he had been conscious. He certainly would have struggled, but there is no evidence of defensive injuries on the hands or fingers, nor are there any injuries on the face that would have indicated that he, in turn, had to be struck by the one or two assailants who would have been fighting with him. An unconscious or dazed condition could have been induced by the application of a drug such as chloroform or ether, or any of the general anesthetic agents that are readily available, none of which would remain within the body long after death, or by a slight blow to the head. The latter possibility is quite likely as there was a small area of superficial scalp hemorrhage on the inside toward the right base of the scalp, and no other head injuries.

Dr. Wecht, therefore, was led to the conclusion that Chen was a victim of homicide, and that his death was caused by being dropped from an upper floor of the fire escape while unconscious.

After returning from Taiwan, Dr. Wecht directed the recommendations summarized below to the government of Taiwan. First and foremost of these is a call for a continuing active investigation into Chen's death. Prior to his departure from Taiwan, during his meeting with the premier of the Republic of China, Yun-suan Sun, Wecht had been assured that this would be done. At that time, Premier Sun stated that the investigation of Chen's death was still open, that the minister of justice had instructed the district attorney to continue investigating the case, and that if new evidence came up it would be evaluated.

Recommendation 1. It is recommended that a vigorous investigation of Dr. Chen's death be continued until these uncertainties have been removed or substantially reduced.

Recommendation 2. It is recommended that all of the available information relating to this case, such as tape recordings, transcripts, and statements of witnesses be made public, with names and sensitive details deleted.

Recommendation 3. It is recommended that in addition to the continuing investigation by the prosecutor's office, an independent commission with nongovernmental membership be established to review all circumstances surrounding Dr. Chen's death and the procedures that were followed in its initial investigations.

Recommendation 4. It is recommended that any person who is questioned by the Taiwan Garrison General Headquarters in the future be permitted to have a lawyer or another witness present during the entire interrogation.

Recommendation 5. It is recommended that, for humanitarian reasons, the government of the Republic of China help to alleviate the financial burden on Su-jen Chen by making payments to her that will help her to raise her one-year-old son, Eric, in a home free from financial stress.

Recommendation 6. It is recommended that a high official of the government of the Republic of China arrange a public visit to Dr. Chen's father and mother to express formally the government's sympathy for their deep personal loss and the government's regrets that this tragedy could have occurred in Taiwan.

Recommendation 7. It is recommended that the government of the Republic of China strive to ensure that all of its citizens can express their views openly in the United States without jeopardiziig their freedom to reenter and leave Taiwan or endangering their personal safety while visiting there.

These recommendations, together with a report of findings made by Dr. Wecht, were presented to Richard M. Cyert, President of Carnegie-Mellon University, who had authorized the trip, and who, in turn, forwarded them to the president of the Republic of China, Chiang Ching-Kuo. High government officials in Taiwan have indicated that several of these recommendations are being implemented. In a statement made to Taiwanese newspapers, the Taiwan Garrison Command indicated that their interrogation procedures will be modified so that, in the future, interviews may be freely declined. And, if a person accepts the interview, he may choose the time and place; interviews in a small room would be avoided in favor of talks in public places, possibly in the presence of friends or relatives. Furthermore, if the person being interviewed cares to bring a lawyer, "the security authority will also consider his wishes." The Garrison Command has also stated that legal measures would be taken against Taiwanese citizens living abroad only if they join organizations whose aims are in direct violation of the constitution or if they actually commit seditious acts. Critical statements made overseas by Taiwanese citizens should not affect the issuance of entry or exit permits.

In the meantime, the official investigation of Chen's death continues. A police task force charged with probing the death has recently been enlarged to include experts in medicine, law, and criminal affairs. And, according to the chief prosecutor of the case, the investigating force is now officially considering the possibility that Chen was murdered.

More than six months after his death, Chen's funeral was held in Taipei on January 7, 1982. Negotiations between Chen's father and the Taiwanese government resulted in a low-key, nonpolitical funeral. The government reportedly promised to support public contributions to pay the funeral expenses, on the condition that no anti-Kuomintang demonstrations occurred. To date, approximately $20,000 has been collected. Although funds collected in excess of the expenses are to be turned over to Chen's widow, the Taiwanese government has not agreed to compensate her directly because, the officials say, such payments could be construed as an admission of guilt.

REFERENCES

1. "Professor Chen Goes Home," *Newsweek*, August 3, 1981, p. 49; "How Did Chen Die?," *Asiaweek*, October 16, 1981, p. 34.
2. Ralph Clough, *Island China*, 1978, p. 35.
3. "How Did Chen Die?," *Asiaweek*, October 16, 1981, p. 43.
4. Clough, *op. cit.*, p. 66.
5. *Asiaweek*, July 11, 1980.

3. Death by Hanging

Bernard J. Ficarra, M.D., Sc.D., Ph.D., LL.D., J.D.

> Death hath ten thousand several doors for men to take their exits.
>
> John Webster, *The Duchess of Malfi*, Act IV, Scene 2

The love of life and the fear of death have been topics of the written and spoken word since the existence of man. Of the two love of life is the one taken more for granted. Fear of death is usually only recognized when people are confronted with its grim finality. Their attitude toward death has been expressed in many ways; and often the manner in which death approaches has altered the observer's response to it. For example, the time of life death reaps its harvest may serve to augment or diminish the surliness of its presence. The ancient scribe, Seneca (4 B.C.–65 A.D.), expressed this in the following way in *Hercules Oetaeus*: "Death is a punishment to some, to others a gift, and to many a favor."

In modern times, the subject of death is usually avoided during normal interaction. Yet, denying, ignoring, and evading its reality has noto abolished it, and the current resurrection of discussion on the topic may be seen as an inevitable, consequence of the current global sociopolitical upheavals.

The melancholic political intransigiency in Northern Ireland has revived discussion about capital punishment by hanging in the British Isles. It has been suggested as a deterrant to violent actions by the Irish. Controversy about this is to be anticipated. It is basic to the issue that any social program, contemplated or instituted, that may be hoped to stem the rise of or curtail violent behavior will have both its proponents and opponents.

The sudden rise in number of suicide by hanging has been cited in the daily press, scientific writings, lay magazines, and other media reports The increasing recurrence of the phenomenon especially among teenagers as a sought-after method of self-destruction is alarming.

The motives behind death by hanging, when studied scientifically and statistically, may be categorized into four groups:

1. instituted as a punishment for crimes against the nation, state, or a fellow citizen
2. as a means of voluntary suicide
3. used as a murder weapon
4. accidental during eroticism.

JUDICIAL HANGING

Anglo-Saxon law stipulated that the method of executing a criminal was to be hanging. Executions in Great Britain and Ireland ceased in 1964, when the death penalty was abolished. The recent rise in advocates for capital punishment has reawakened interest in the modalities employed by nations and states to accomplish this purpose.

Some insights into judicial hanging have been recorded by a member of an English family whose name has been on the "short Home Office list of qualified executioners" for the first forty-six years of the twentieth century[1]. Some highlights of this history have been incorporated into the following discussion.

There is no definitive explanation as to why any person should elect to become a professional executioner. To be certain, a man who selects this position must be an entity unto himself with personal, mental, social, and other characteristics that separate him from almost everyone else in human society. One trait, however, has been emphasized. "Vengeance is not and cannot be any aspect of an executioner's participation."[1].

Either through apprenticeship or actual schooling at certain prisons (called "gaols" in England), the historic science of hanging is taught. Associated with the technique are instructions in supplementary rituals given to the neophyte. For example, in the first decade of this century, it was a practice to fly a black flag to show that a prisoner had been executed. "By order of the Home Secretary, a bell was tolled instead—but this solemnity, too, was later discontinued."[1].

Judicial hanging, as perfected in Great Britain, required that the executioner prepare the setting with precise calculations. Familiarity with the penal equipment was necessary in order to master the technique and obtain the maximum speed. Pierrepont stated that: "My father could dispatch a man in the time it took the prison clock to strike eight—leading him from his cell on the first stroke and having him suspended dead on the rope by the last stroke. That seemed a very worthy intermediate ambition for me.''[1].

Curiosity demands an explanation of the head-covering placed over the condemned person. The white cap, which is erroneously referred to and depicted as black in films or television productions, ''has been used in British executions from the later days of batch-strangulation in public, long before the introduction of the long drop designed to sever the cervical vertebrae and cause spontaneous death. Its original purpose was to mask the contortions of slow strangulation, which were considered too horrible even for the ghoulish British public to witness, although the logic that public executions were a public deterrent against crime might have been followed strictly by exposing the ultimate horror in order to achieve the maximum deterrence''[1].

A mercy to the condemned victim as well, the cap prevented the prisoner from judging the exact moment the lever was pulled. The routine procedure is to slip the cap (a spacious white cotton bag) over the head. The noose is adjusted immediately over the cap. The practical advantage of this is that, ''with the rope holding the cap, no sudden up-draught caused by the drop can lift the cap from the face.''[1].

The presence of press representatives at executions was standard. ''When an execution was bungled, the newspapers had no hesitation in reporting it.''[1]. As a result of criticism in newspaper reports, the Home Office initiated research into then-current methods of judicial hanging. This culminated in ''the preparation of a standard table of drops, which was recommended in 1888''[1]. The table was a simplified extension of the formula:

$$\frac{\text{1260 foot pounds}}{\text{weight of prisoner in pounds}} = \text{length of the recommended drop in feet}$$

> A master executioner is responsible for every detail of his craft. He has to come to his own decision on the length of the drop based on the Home Office table, varied by his own experience, and adjusted to the weight of the prisoner, his height, his age, and an estimate of the musculature and tensile strength of his neck. This nuchal strength can be varied by such circumstances as a recent attempt at suicide by cutting the throat, not an uncommon occurrence following crimes of sudden passion[1].

After the victim's body is hanging in the pit, the execution house is closed until nine o'clock A.M., when the executioner and his assistant withdraw the body. The executed person is released from the rope and removed to a pathology room. All other execution equipment is taken from the scaffold area by the assistant. Simultaneously, official notices are posted at the prison gates, certifying that the death sentence has been carried out.

All executed miscreants are usually subjected to a postmortem examination. Special attention is given to the vertebral column. A perfect execution by hanging is reported in the autopsy protocol as instantaneous death due to "fracture dislocation of the second and third cervical vertebrae with severed spinal column"[1].

In order to produce this result, it is necessary to apply the noose properly. When Pierrepoint was in training to become an executioner, he took instruction at the Pentonville Prison in London. His first exercise was in applying the noose correctly.

Draw it firm and tight with the free end of the rope emerging from the metal eye just under the left jawbone. There is no knot. That fancy cowboy coil of a 'hangman's noose (knot)' is something we abandoned to the Americans a hundred years ago. In Britain, the rope runs free through a pear-shaped metal eye woven into the rope's end, and the operative part of the noose is covered with soft wash-leather. Always adjust it to the left, because with the pull of the drop the noose gyrates a quarter-circle clockwise and the tug of the rope finishes under the chin. This motion throws the neck back and breaks the spinal column, separating it at about the third vertebra of the neck. Adjust it on the right and it gyrates to the back of the neck, throwing the head forward, not breaking the neck, eventually killing by suffocation[1].

Judicial hanging became a streamlined, meticulous procedure, with all the exactitude of a surgical operation.

The executioner and his assistant wait outside the condemned man's cell, with the chief officer and second officer detailed to conduct the prisoner to the execution chamber. On a signal given by the sheriff, they enter, and the executioner pinions the prisoner's arms behind his back. He is escorted to the drop with one officer on either side. The sheriff, the prison governor, and the medical officer enter the execution chamber directly by another door.

The prisoner is placed on the drop at a marked spot so that his feet are directly across the division of the trap doors. The executioner places a white cap over the prisoner's head and puts the noose round his neck, while the assistant pinions his legs. When the executioner sees that all is ready he pulls the lever. The medical officer at once proceeds to the pit and examines the prisoner to see that life is extinct. The shed is then locked and the body hangs for one hour. The inquest is held the same morning[1].

In the London area, a postmortem was mandatory. Outside of the city and its environs, an autopsy study was not always compulsory.

An historical review shows that, in 1832, there were two hundred and twenty offences deemed punishable by death in Great Britain.

By 1837, the number was reduced to fifteen. In 1861, the death penalty was restricted to the offences of murder, treason, piracy with violence, and arson in the Sovereign's vessels, arsenals, or dockyards.[1].

In 1938, a House of Commons motion suspending capital punishment for peacetime crimes for an experimental period of five years was carried, but ignored, and in the next year a similarly phrased bill was defeated. In 1948, an amendment to the Criminal Justice

Bill advocating a five-year suspension of capital punishment was passed narrowly in the House of Commons, but was defeated in the House of Lords. The bill was passed without it. But, in the interim period between the votes, an abnormal number of reprieves was granted by the Home Secretary. As a result of this activity, a Royal Commission was set up in 1949 to consider whether or not capital punishment for murder should be limited or modified[1].

In England

the outcry against the execution of Ruth Ellis in July 1955, after conviction for the murder of a lover who had discarded her, was the last great sentimental protest against capital punishment. Afterwards, the imposition of the death sentence was restricted to a narrow range of crimes. These were murder by shooting or explosives, murder done in furtherance of theft, murder of a police officer or prison officer on duty, or effected in order to escape from legal custody. Later, even these offences ceased to be classed as capital murder. There has been no judicial hanging in England since 1964[1].

Reflecting upon his twenty-five years as an executioner, Pierrepont writes:

I believed with all my heart that I was carrying out a public duty. I conducted each execution [there were about 400 in all] with great care and a clear conscience. I never allowed myself to get involved with the death penalty controversy. I now sincerely hope that no man is ever called upon to carry out another execution in my country. I have come to the conclusion that executions solve nothing and are only an antiquated relic of a primitive desire for revenge which takes the easy way and hands over the responsibility for revenge to other people. It is said to be a deterrent. I cannot agree. There have been murders since the beginning of time and we shall go on looking for deterrents until the end of time. If death were a deterrent, I might be expected to know. All the men and women whom I have faced at that final moment convince me that in what I have done I have not prevented a single murder[1].

The author-executioner continues in a moral key:

I may add that there is never at any execution the situation where an unwilling executioner is ordered to take an action which he dare not refuse. This would . . . parallel the defense offered by some Germans accused of war crimes, such as [those] convicted of killing Royal Air Force escaped prisoners of war. Their defense was that they were given orders which it would have been contrary to their oath of loyalty to refuse. No executioner is appointed under sealed orders to perform any execution as directed by his superiors. He is first asked if he is available to do that particular duty involving a particular prisoner on a specific date. If he says he is not available, the matter ends, as far as he is concerned. He is an officer of the state, but his rigid obedience extends only to the duties he voluntarily opts to do[1].

Current sociopolitical events in England have raised the notion of a return to the gallows. However,

One of the largest Conservative majorities in modern parliamentary history voted against bringing back the gallows in Britain. Prime Minister Margaret Thatcher, who has supported restoration of the death penalty for acts of terrorism and other violent crimes, freed members of her party to vote their conscience. Public opinion polls showed strong sentiment in favor of hanging, but British institutions concerned with its legal and moral ramifications generally opposed it. In the death penalty debate, the government official responsible for Northern Ireland affairs carried much weight. He said the Irish Republican Army would try to benefit from the use of capital punishment by creating martyrs. A Roman Catholic member of parliament from Northern Ireland said the death penalty would play into the hands of the terrorists[2].

SUICIDE AS A GENERAL PHENOMENON

The social dimensions of suicide are often overshadowed by the tragic personal consequences that attend the act. In Ancient Greece, the antisocial nature of suicide was implied via the prerequisite that the person contemplating it would first have to secure permission from the senate. Another social characteristic of it is that suicidal persons seem to gravitate to one another. It also at times seems to be contagious. "The reported deaths by suicide of several students in a New Jersey school and of nearly one thousand people in Guyana, call attention both to the contagious element in suicide, and to the questions of the social significance of suicide"[3].

Sharing in the suicide of a beloved friend, relative, or celebrity for some people is a social expression of sympathy. "A sense of sharing in the suicide of someone famous or of identifying one's suicide with a sociopolitical cause enables some persons to feel their deaths have a societal meaning it would lack otherwise."[3]. Studies have indicated that, indeed, after the death by suicide of famous people, many other suicides follow. When Socrates was forced to drink the cup of hemlock, many of his students did the same. And oriental cultures even sanction the pursuit of suicide, family style.

Western civilizations have branded suicide with dishonor. Denying proper burial to the corpse of a suicide or imposing fines or imprisonment on anyone surviving a suicide attempt has been common practices at various times.

Retrospective studies indicate that a great majority, approximately two-thirds, of persons who eventually commit suicide have a history of prior attempts at it. Some authorities on thanatology contend that suicide is a symptom of mental aberration. Mental illness is, indeed, terminated in the cases of some unfortunate individuals by voluntary suicide. In general, the suicidal person is one who has been mentally or physically ill or has suffered a deep loss or grave disappointment, or someone who has been treated shabbily in either a real or imagined manner[4].

Since the 1960s, suicides among the young have been steadily increasing[5]. Suicide has risen statistically, becoming the fourth-ranking cause of death among 15- to 19-year-old adolescents in 1974[6]. Between 1980 and 1985, a doubling of the rate of adolescents' hospital admissions for suicide attempts has been reported[7]. Studying forty adolescent patients under psychiatric therapy following suicide attempts, a researcher arrived at the following conclusions:

1. All were psychiatrically ill before the suicide attempt;
2. The most common diagnoses were those of depressive disorders and substance-abuse disorders on the clinical psychiatric syndrome axis; and,
3. Borderline personality disorder on the personality and developmental disorder axis[8].

A composite clinical collage typifies the suicidal patient as a drug abuser with a borderline personality disorder and a major depressive disorder. Girls attempt suicide in greater numbers than do the boys.

The most prominent personality characteristics associated with suicide attempts by these adolescents were a tendency to react severely to a loss, poorly controlled rage, and impulsivity. Suicide attempts by adolescents should be taken seriously by the physician. It necessitates a thorough search for a possible underlying pathological condition[8].

Youthful death is recalled dramatically in Shakespearean drama. The unnecessary deaths of Romeo and Juliet emphasize the overwhelming tragedy of the mistaken death of Juliet and the voluntary suicide of hapless Romeo. A philosophical epithet was whispered by the confused Romeo to the apparently dead Juliet:

> "Ah, dear Juliet,
> Why art thou yet so fair? Shall I believe
> That unsubstantial death is amorous"[9].

Professional persons are not exempt from the suicidal horror. A formal evaluation was made of an epidemic of suicide among physicians who had been put on probation by a state board of medical examiners.

The disciplinary mode of the board is expressed in its powers of probation. When a physician in the specific state is found culpable of professional misconduct of sufficient weight to merit probation, his or her license to practice is suspended and immediately reinstated, generally for a probationary period of ten years[10].

Commenting on their conclusions, the psychiatrists brought forth the fact that the most obvious single common element among these physicians was a serious psychopathological condition that recurrs throughout their active professional lives. Secondarily, a prominent corollary was the abuse of alcohol and other mind-altering drugs[10].

Historical medical data disclosed that

professional status was of singular importance to these physicians. This goal was embodied by professional achievement and the personal acceptance by their physician peers. These goals were of such importance that they were pursued at the expense of positive family relationship and community networks. While some of these probationers experienced financial difficulties that probably contributed to their stress, financial problems were not perceived by the survivors or by the study group as having a direct causal relationship to their deaths. All of the physicians were migrants to the state. In most instances, their domestic and social lives were characterized by a severe sense of isolation[10].

Modern suicidologists classify suicide as either interpersonal or intrapersonal. Interpersonal suicide victims make frequent threats and attempts to kill themselves. They possess emotional liability, ill-defined suicide plans, and a fairly clear idea of how their crisis might be resolved. Intrapersonal suicide victims are less open in showing their suicidal drives. They are withdrawn personalities rather than emotional. These intrapersonal unfortunate people show clearly formulated plans, but have no solutions other than suicide to end their crisis. Both types find their origin in the loss of a valued relative or friend, an intangible source, or loss in self-esteem. The intrapersonal victim is less accessible and more difficult to reach and to help[11].

Suicide is the last resort when all other avenues for the resolution of crises have been traveled. Behavior patterns leading to intentional suicide are viewed by the misguided stress victims as a final answer to their quandry. The crisis theory in psychiatry dictates that a person contemplating suicide is receptive to assistance during a period of crisis. It is implied that persons in a state of mental disquiet may be amenable to the acceptance of medical advice[12]. The physician often can assess a suicidal person's psychological status quickly and easily. An immediate professional evaluation can determine the course of treatment to be followed, whether inside or out of the hospital. Psychiatric assistance is not to be denied to the crisis-burdened patient[11]. These suicide-oriented are hungry for love, lonely for appreciation, and often misunderstood.

SUICIDE BY HANGING

Voluntary death by hanging was stamped with ignominy when Judas Ischariot hanged himself after betraying His Lord for thirty pieces of silver. Since then, suicidal hanging has carried an evil connotation. Such a mode of death is in someways sadder than death itself, another example of humanity batting its ephemeral wings against an impregnable void.

Love suicides have been romanticized in the cinema, in drama, on television, and even in the comic strips. Young people in particular seem to be attracted to suicide by hanging.

One survey indicated that 60 percent of high school students had the thought of suicide at least once in their short life. Now, many boys and girls in primary school are committing suicide; over 100 a year under fourteen years of age have been recorded with ten times that number trying it[3].

In Japan young people probe into the psychologic aspects of suicide as not being an abnormal interest. The statistical fact is that "purposeless suicides for the sake of suicide are on the rise. Three desires seem to be in the minds of young suicides: the desire to kill, the desire to be killed, and the desire to die"[18].

It appears that the younger generations are not realistic about the finality of suicide. Few young people recognize the permanency of death as the grim reaper of life. "Few children have seen the death of a household pet or any animal at close quarters. So, without fear, they lightheartedly leap from life to death as simply as crossing a street"[13]. Thus, through suicide they have made a covenant with death.

Suicidal hanging is earmarked characteristically as causing death by compression of the anatomic airway and the blood vessels in the neck. The body weight, by sagging, produces the slow compression that eventuates in death through suffocation, unconsciousness, and asphyxia. The sagging, dependent weight of the body is sufficient to choke and strangle the victim, but is inadequate to transect the cervical spinal cord, as in a judicial hanging where the "body drop" intensifies the line of cervical force.

In suicidal hanging, all kinds of material may be used to make a noose, in addition to a rope or a segment of clothesline. Belts, electric wires, towels, clothing, ties, and other unusual items have been discovered around suicide victims' necks. These ligatures are usually located above the thyroid cartilage, going behind the ears, with a knot finding its resting place in the vicinity of the external occipital protuberance (the inion). Hanging by the full weight of the body causes death from the prompt bilateral compression of the carotid arteries. After death has supervened, the face is pale, looking similar to cases of exsanguination.

When the lower extremities support the body or the ligature is placed around the neck asymmetrically, immediate arterial compression does not occur, nor is tracheal collapse instantaneous. Since the point of suspension is not at the inion, but either to the right or to the left of it, compression is gradual. Progressive occlusion is slow, with collapse of the veins first and arterial brain circulation being diminished slowly thereafter. Thus petechial hemorrhages are seen on the face and in the conjunctivae.

The standing position is that most frequently chosen in suicidal hanging. Next in frequency is standing on a chair and kicking it after a ligature has been attached overhead. Suicidal hanging with knees bent after two ropes have been tied about the neck going to the right and left has been recorded less frequently. Many esoteric positions have been tried by successful suicides not to mention others who were not so successful.

HANGING AS A MURDER WEAPON

An essential function of coroners and medical examiners is to properly and scientifically classify all deaths they are called upon to investigate. Officially, there are five classifications: natural, accidental, suicidal, homicidal, and undetermined. Among these, it is sometimes most difficult to distinguish murder from suicide[4]. This is especially a concern of police authorities in hanging cases, which are almost always classified as suicides. Murder by hanging is not, for example, one of the methods used by organized crime. However, it *is* a means of causing harm in certain Oriental cultures and among various island inhabitants.

In order to differentiate suicidal hanging from murder, it is well to remember that death by strangulation results from asphyxiation. Body weight, as in death by judicial hanging, does not play a major rôle in this pathophysiologic suicidal mechanism. Hence, strangulation by a noose can be the result of either suicide or homicide. In both cases, the carotid arteries and jugular veins are compressed. The lumina of the vertebral arteries in their bony protection remain viable and opened. This vertebral arterial blood supply produces facial congestion and petechial hemorrhages on visible mucosal surfaces.

After death, certain clues are detectable that can be used to distinguish homicidal from suicidal hanging. Among the telltale signs are:

1. The ligating material, such as rope, when knotted anteriorly, may have been tied by someone other than the deceased;
2. When the length of the rope ends are equal, it is usually suicide;
3. In homicide, the ends of the rope or other ligating material usually are unequal, meaning that one segment of the material is longer than the other beyond the tied knot;
4. The victim of homicide has a rope or other material ligated around the neck once and then tightened. Death by hanging would not result because the knot would loosen and inadequate pressure would be present to cause compression of the airway and the arteries: body weight, with the onset of unconsciousness, would liberate the neck from its noose;
5. In suicidal hanging, the knots are very tight or the ligature is doubled (twice or more around the neck); and,
6. During a murder by manual strangulation made to look like a suicidal hanging, fingernail scratch marks may be present on the neck from when the deceased fought to release the pressure on his or her neck.

There have been instances where a person has been murdered via manual strangulation. Death results from asphyxia. In order to mimic suicide by hanging, the miscreant then places a rope around the victim's neck. An examination of the deceased will show hemorrhage in the soft tissues of the neck, especially in the sternohyoid, sternothyroid, and omohyoid muscles. In addition to the hemorrhage, a fracture of the hyoid bone, thyroid cartilage, or laryngeal cartilages may be present. Because manual strangulation is not conducive to the application of bilateral equal pressure when the victim is struggling, compression of the airway and vascular channels is incomplete, resulting in facial congestion and mucosal petechiae. Often, the medical examiner discerns fingernail scratches or skin indentations in the neck region as an indication of the victim's attempt to release the attacker's manual pressure.

Those who are attuned to professional wrestling are familiar with the "sleeper hold" applied to the neck in the form of a headlock. This hold can result in neurogenic shock. The mechanism is mediated through the carotid sinus stimulation reaction known as Czermak's reflex (named after Johann Nepomuk Czermak, 1828–1873, an Austrian otolaryngologist and physiologist). Compression of the neck can stimulate the carotid sinus to such a degree that death occurs. Manual strangulation can cause this type of death. Carotid sinus death is not revealed by any positive pathologic finding at autopsy.

ACCIDENTAL HANGING

Add sexual perversion to the woes of mankind. When men or women try to improve on nature's biological methods, they not only become frustrated, but worse, act unnaturally, and usually to their own detriment. Any sexual behavior that strays from the confines of normal physiological compatibility is considered to be a perversion. At one time, deviation from the normal sexual profile was regarded as a form of mental illness. Present-day social attitudes are more liberal in this matter. Nonetheless, pygmalionism, narcissism, sadism, necrophilia, sodomy, tribadism, and pederasty are abnormal sexual practices.

One may add to the list another deviation, described by the Marquis de Sade: self-induced asphyxia as a means of ejaculatory gratification in the form of masturbation[15]. The majority of persons indulging in this form of eroticism are men. A common underlying psychosomatic format is discerned in these people with regard to age, gender, physical attributes, and mental orientation. Many of the men who pursue autoerotic asphyxial maneuvers are transvestites.

Unfortunately, the intended erotic pleasure can result in unintentional self-destruction by hanging. Although autoerotic asphyxial deaths are not a daily occurrence, the current laxity in the general social attitude toward sexual modus operandi augurs for the future increase in reported instances of this phenomenon.

Medicolegal knowledge of this aspect of human behavior is necessary, because clandestine sexual activities can and do result in death, especially in the case of autoerotic asphyxia. The manner of death here initially points to suicide, but in most instances the occurrences are accidental. From the viewpoint of the family member who may claim insurance benefits, the difference between death by suicide or by misadventure can be readily appreciated. Voluntary suicide by hanging has a different compensatory value than involuntary, accidental suicide.

Scientific studies on autoerotic asphyxial deaths have elucidated various diagnostic features that help to distinguish suicide from an accidental death occurring during unusual sexual maneuvers or gymnastics. The psychiatric, psychological, and medical literature on this subject is not voluminous, but is nonetheless quite excellent [23,24,25]. All the studies have found the accident victims, though possessing various character traits, to be loners, isolationists, and depressed, with an abnormal fixation on death [19,20,21].

Investigation into this medical curiosity—which has begun to occur more frequently than is realized—indicates that it is nothing new. The induction of a transitory asphyxiation via the compression of the carotid blood vessels in the neck as a means of sexual arousement is a practice documented by anthropologists to have been performed for centuries.[22]. Eskimos are known to choke one another as part of their sexual repetoire and normal love activity. It is not unusual for Eskimo children to suspend themselves by the neck as a routine play procedure[23].

For the physician and others necessarily involved in medicolegal matters, the following clues are graphic signs that differentiate suicide from an autoerotic accident:

1. The finding of asphyxia resulting from strangulation via a ligature or strangulation by hanging;
2. Evidence that death was not intended, based upon the position of the body or the presence of protective gear such as neck padding (towel, shirt, trousers);
3. Signs of sexual activity (masturbation) or perversion (transvestism);
4. Indication of prior similar episodes of abnormal human behavior (marks on rafters or doors);
5. Absence of a history of a specific tendency toward suicide, ideation in this direction, or suicidal behavior formula; and,
6. Asphyxia due to strangulation by ligature and suffocation, which is more common than strangulation by hanging, causing an accidental death[17,22].

When propelled by concupiscence, the unfortunate person with autoerotic propensities does not suspect that death lurks nearby. Sexual gratification via constriction of the neck is inherently perilous because of the ever-present threat of asphyxiation. This sensual pursuit involves young men who practice it as a form of sadomasochism, sexual fantasy, or both. Often, the man is a transvestite who wears female apparel. Associated with the eroticism is constriction of the genitalia with ligatures (referred to as bondage). Death is not intended, which is indicated by the incomplete suspension of the body (feet still on the floor), or the proximity of the body to furniture (usually a chair) which would allow a release of the neck constriction. Involuntary death is further substantiated by some evidence that the individual has performed these abnormal acts previously. The give away signs are notations found in a personal diary, a history of similar deviant behavior, conversations with friends or neighbors on this topic, and physical signs of grooves (or other markings) in ceiling rafters, doors, or furniture from rope, cord, wire, or other ligature material[22].

Another indicator that death was not intended is based upon the detailed preparation of the bondage technique. Additional substantiating findings include the presence of mirrors, and photography equipment for reviewing the genitalia.

The outstanding visible sign that leads to the conclusion of an accidental death is "the protection of the neck . . . padding between the neck and the ligature"[22].

Autopsy protocols do not point to any specific cause of death indigenous to this mode of dying. The pathological anatomical findings are nonspecific but are similar to those reported in death by asphyxiation in general. The identifiable pathological entities are pulmonary edema, visceral congestion, and petechial hemorrhages. Sometimes, the victim of autoerotic asphyxia takes drugs or imbibes alcohol prior to the deviant episode. Toxicological studies will identify the alcohol or the ingested drug (most often a barbiturate).

Death via autoerotic asphyxiation has some major legal ramifications, the most significant of which in civilian life concerns insurance claims[24,25]. Most life insurance contracts have limitations or exceptions on coverage when death occurs by suicide. Certain life insurance policies have an increased payment under an accidental death clause. Other commercial accident insurance contracts specify payment of the face value amount to be paid for accidental death and lesser amounts for accidental dismemberment or other disabilities that are accident related [22,26].

The legal definition of accident has not always been the same. Variations have been stated legally in different court decisions. Among these are that an accident is:

1. Any event that takes place without the foresight or expectation of the person acted upon or affected thereby;
2. A happening or coming by chance or without design; casual, fortuitous, taking place unexpectedly, unintentionally, or out of the usual course of events; and,
3. Something unforeseen, unexpected, or extraordinary[27].

The word, accident, is derived from the Latin verb, *accidere*, signifying "fall upon," "befall," "happen," "chance," or "unexpected." In an etymological appraisal, anything that happens can be interpreted as an accident. In its more formal accepted meaning, accident is defined as a fortuitous circumstance, event, or happening. It is an event happening wholly or partly through human agency, an event which, under the circumstances, is unusual and unexpected by the person to whom it happens [28]. An accident is an untoward occurrence in the usual course of events[29]. It may be without known or an assignable cause[30]. In its proper use, the term excludes negligence[31].

There is no standardization in the opinion of insurance carriers as to whether autoerotic asphyxial death qualifies as an accident. Most insurance companies would not pay the beneficiary without a thorough investigation. Some insurance carriers may accept the manner of death as listed on the death certificate without an in-depth scrutiny. Autoerotic asphyxial death, by its very circumstance, arouses a great deal of suspicion. Insurers, therefore, would not pay out a double indemnity, for example, without a minute evaluation of the mode of death, even if it was listed as natural, undetermined, or accidental[22].

When a person is in the military service, and death results from any autoerotic behavior, a more clearly defined set of rules and regulations prevail. "The payment of survivors benefits is connected intimately with the determination made in the line-of-duty investigation"[22]. "If the injury or death was incurred as a result of erratic or reckless conduct or other deliberate course of conduct without regard for personal safety, or the safety of others, it was incurred not in the line of duty, but was due to misconduct."[22,32] If a member of the armed forces was mentally unsound at the time of his or her injury, disease, or death, he or she cannot be held responsible for his or her acts, and a determination in his or her favor must be made, unless the mental unsoundness was due to his or her own misconduct[33].

Even if the manner of death in autoerotic asphyxia is determined to be accidental, it has been stated

> that the deceased did not intend to take his life, but deliberately asphyxiated himself to the verge of unconsciousness for the purpose of sexual gratification. Under these circumstances, the individual's activities could be regarded as erratic or reckless conduct or other deliberate course of conduct, without regard for personal safety, constituting gross neglect, and therefore [death] was incurred not in the line of duty but was due to his own misconduct[22].

AUTOPSY AFTER SUICIDE

In a dazed and distraught condition, a man decided that his suicide—staged to appear like an accident—would allow his widow to collect a double indemnity from their insurance company. The autopsy eventually unmasked the suicide.

As many as 20 percent of any physician's patients may be depressed, and depression is a major factor leading to suicide. So widespread is self-destruction that there has been created an endowed study that "will attempt to obtain accurate, relevant information through a psychological autopsy concerning deaths by suicide. It consists of an interview with the next of kin conducted by a psychiatrist"[34].

Autopsy analysis is an indispensable keystone in the medicolegal armamentarian. Recognition of its acceptance is verified by the program instituted with acclaim by the National Institute of Justice, a program designed to improve the investigation of deaths from other than natural causes. The project aims to perfect procedures to assist coroners, medical examiners, and law enforcement personnel in their investigation of medicolegal deaths or any suspicious death. Many experienced medicolegal experts believe that one-third of all deaths reported annually are suspicious in nature and require a very thorough autopsy[35].

In general, an autopsy

> reveals what is to be seen. It does not provide the information concerning how the death occurred. The findings made at an autopsy may be interpreted quite differently under dissimilar circumstances. The autopsy provides answers, but (often) not the answer re-

quested. The autopsy is not synonymous with postmortem examination, as many people think. While essential to the investigation, the autopsy is only a part of the postmortem examination, which includes a wide range of investigatory procedures. The investigation of the scene of death and a critical analysis of the circumstantial factors are important parts of the postmortem examination[36].

As in any medical study, the history of the person involved, whether as a living person or as the subject for a postmortem, is not to be ignored. To underestimate a clinical history or totally ignore it can lead the investigator down the wrong path and to erroneous conclusions. Autopsy findings often are elusive or misleading. Without an adequate history, the puzzle can be distorted, or significant guiding information can remain concealed. In the necropsy room, the medicolegalist may witness the final result of disease and the failure of the human body to solve its problems. However, the knowledge to be gained through each individual autopsy is limited. Just as there is an obvious limit to what one can learn about normal business transactions from a daily visit to the bankruptcy court, one must remember that the autopsy findings are not the oracle at Delphi[37].

CONCLUSION

The topic of hanging is not for genteel discourse at social gatherings. A better knowledge of this phenomenon, however, has become medically necessary by dint of its growing frequency in modern society. The confusion often attendant upon this usually surreptitious event must be unravelled by those attuned to medicolegal problems. Suicide by hanging is becoming more common with the passage of time. In certain jurisdictions, it is looked upon as a criminal offense. When capital punishment was in force, judicial hanging was a legal method that some state authorities used for putting criminals to death. A reawakened controversy on capital punishment has provoked a renewed assessment of judicial hanging in some European nations.

Life is precious. When it is prematurely extinguished, it brings a sadness without equal. When death results from hanging, the sorrow is accentuated. Lethal hanging leaves an ineradicable, terrible memory, and hanging as self-annihilation is becoming a readily adopted alternative to life in our frustrated, thanatophilic society. The Latin poet, Juvenal (60?–140?) wrote in *Satires* (X,356): "Pray first for a sound mind in a sound body." This advice, if followed, may well provide us with one of our best defenses against suicide.

REFERENCES

1. Pierrepoint, Albert, "Executioner: Pierrepoint." Sixth Impression. Hodder and Stoughton Ltd., Great Britain, 1977.

2. No author. "M.P.'s say no to new gallows by wide margin." *New York Times* July 17, 1983.

3. Hendin, H., "A saner policy on suicide." *Psychology Today*, 115, 1979.
4. "Suicide in childhood." Editorial in *JAMA*, Feb. 20, 1904. Recounted in *JAMA*, vol. 24, 8, February 23, 1979.
5. Hollinger, C. P., "Adolescent suicide: An epidemiological study of recent trends." *Am. Jour. Psychiatry*, vol. 61, 4, 1978, 204, 210.
6. Murphy, G. K., "Sudden deaths in adolescents." *Jour. Pediatrics*, vol. 61, 4, 1978, 204, 210.
7. Schneer, H., Perlstein, A., and Brozobsky, M., "Hospitalized suicidal adolescents: Two generations." *Jour. Am. Academy Child Psychiatry*, vol. 14, 6, 1975, 268, 280.
8. Crumley, F., "Adolescent suicide attempts." *JAMA*, vol. 241, 22, June 1, 1979, 2404, 2407.
9. Shakespeare, W., *Romeo and Juliet*, Act V, Scene III, lines 101–103.
10. Crawshaw, R., Bruce, J. Eraker, P., Greenbaum, M., Lindemann, J., and Schmidt, D., "An epidemic of suicide among physicians on probation." *JAMA*, vol. 241, 19, May 16, 1980, 1915, 1917.
11. Ruben, H., "Managing suicidal behavior." *JAMA*, vol. 241, 19, January 19, 1979, 282, 284.
12. Hankoff, L., "Categories of attempted suicide: A longitudinal study." *Am. Jour. Public Health*, vol. 66, 6, 1976, 558, 563.
13. Flinn, Rev. Kevin, "Suicide syndrome." *Columban Mission Magazine*, June-July, 1983, 12, 14.
14. Yong-Myun, Rho., "Murder or suicide?" *New York State Jour. Medicine*, vol. 78, 5, May, 1978, 965, 967.
15. De Sade, Marquis., *The 120 Days of Sodom and Other Writings*. A. Wainhouse, and R. Seaver eds. Grove Press, New York, N.Y., 1966, 488, 685–85.
16. Weinmann, S., "Sexual asphyxia." In *Textbook of Legal Medicine*, O. Prokop ed. Germany: Veb Volk and Gesundheit, 1960.
17. Mant, J. *Forensic Medicine*, Chicago: Year Book Publishing Co., 1960.
18. Van Hecke, W., and Timperman, A. "Hangings as the cause of accidental death in an unusual form of sex perversion." *Annals of Legal Medicine*, vol. 43, 2, 1963, 218, 219.
19. Sterna, J., "Cases of probable suicide in young persons without obvious motivations." *Maine Med. Ass. Jour.*, vol. 44, 5, 1958, 16.
20. Luke, M., "Asphyxial deaths by hanging in New York City, 1964–1965." *Jour. Forensic Sciences*, vol. 12, 4, 1967, 359.
21. Henry, B., "Death during deviant sexual activity." Paper presented at the Annual Meeting of the American Academy of Forensic Sciences, Chicago, Illinois, 1968.
22. Walsh, F., Stahl, III, C., Unger, H., Lilienstern, O., and Stephens, III, R. "Autoerotic asphyxial deaths: A medicolegal analysis of forty-three cases." *Legal Medicine Annual*, 157, 182. New York: Appleton-Century-Crofts, 1977, 157, 182.
23. Freuchen, G., *Book of the Eskimos*. New York: World Publications, 1961, 212.
24. Richardson and Breyfogle., "Medicolegal problems in suicide versus accident." *Annals Internal Medicine*, vol. 25, 3, 1946, 22, 26.
25. Morse, T., "Law and Medicine: Suicide." *JAMA*, vol. 231, 10, 1967, 200, 263.
26. East, B., "Suicide from the medicolegal aspect." *British Medical Journal*, vol. 2, 1, 1932, 241.

27. Brossman, J., "Insurance death by suicide." *New York State Jour. Medicine*, 32, 6, 1932, 976.

28. Black, H. C., *Law Dictionary*, Fourth Edition. St. Paul: West Publishing Company, 1951.

29. Adams, V., Metropolitan Life Insurance Co., 136 Pa. Super. 454, 7 A 2d 544, 547.

30. *Ramsay V. Sullivan Mining Co.*, 51 Idaho 366, 6 P 2d 856, 858.

31. *Dallas Ry. and Terminal Co. V. Allen*, Texas Civ. App., 43 S.W. 2d 165, 170.

32. Department of the Army, Pam. 27–6, paragraph 4, March 17, 1965.

33. Department of the Army, Pam. 27–6, paragraph 12, rules 10 and 11 March 17, 1965.

34. No author. "Physicians suicides to be topic of study." *American Medical News*, American Medical Association, December 19, 1980, 10.

35. Sullivan, J. O., "Justice to set uniform standards for suspicious death probes." *Trial Magazine*, January, 1981, 11.

36. Rho, Y-M., "Forensic pathology in crimes of violence." F.B.I. Law Enforcement Bulletin, vol. 44, 2, October, 1975.

37. Russell, W., (Lord Brain), *Canadian Medical Association Journal*, vol. 83, 6, 1960, 349.

4. Medical Expert Testimony in the Jean Harris Case

A. Bernard Ackerman, M.D.

INTRODUCTION

In this era of intensive peer review within the medical profession, it is quite timely and appropriate to examine the quality and validity of expert scientific testimony in the courtroom. This chapter by a nationally prominent dermatopathologist, A. Bernard Ackerman, M.D., deals with the medical expert testimony in the Jean Harris trial, which took place in late 1980 - early 1981 in Westchester County, New York.

Several forensic pathologists and dermatopathologists testified concerning various aspects of the shooting of Dr. Herman Tarnower by Jean Harris on March 10, 1980. Dr. Ackerman, one of the defense expert witnesses, experienced problems that were new to him and quite different from anything he had ever previously encountered within the private practice or teaching of his medical specialty.

His personal account of this experience is presented with clarity and candor. Contained within the context of one of the most exciting and interesting murder cases in recent years, the discussion in this chapter will be of much interest and practical value to physicians, forensic scientists, and trial attorneys.

The Physician as Expert Witness—Is Peer Review Needed?*

The expert medical witness in our system of jurisprudence enjoys the widest latitude in the range of scientific facts he may testify about. The only requirement for an expert physician to testify in a particular case is that he be found "qualified" in his area of expertise by the trial judge. Usually, proof that the doctor is licensed to practice medicine in the state of venue is sufficient foundation to allow him to testify.

Under our adversary system of justice, each side in the case has an opportunity to cross-examine the witnesses of the opposing side. The purpose of cross-examination is to expose the flaws and weaknesses in the testimony of opposing witnesses. The theory is that out of this often rough-and-tumble confrontation, metaphorically described by an authority on evidence as "the greatest engine for the discovery of truth," the jury will have before it all the relevant facts upon which a reasoned and just decision can be arrived at. Thus, by legal standards, the fairness of a trial in which scientific-medical issues are at stake is met when the lawyers for each party have had the opportunity for full, unimpeded cross-examination.

The point I address in this article is whether such legal machinery for a full and fair inquiry is, by itself, adequate to assure that lay juries not be egregiously misled when medical "facts" are erroneously testified to by a medical witness. I also address the question of whether or not the medical profession should concern itself in a more systematic way with the conduct of its members when they testify as expert witnesses. In short, is the giving of expert medical testimony so proper a professional activity that it ought not be subject to peer review, as are virtually all other medical activities of importance? Last, I address the issue of the medical witness who becomes a partisan witness. Does such partisanship impair the truth-finding function of juries?

I was one of eight pathologists who were called as expert witnesses in the case of *The People of the State of New York v. Jean S. Harris*. Almost nine full days of the fifty days of the trial (nearly 20 percent) were devoted to issues of cutaneous histology. I have read the transcript of the testimony of all of the pathologists, and this article summarizes what I perceive to be the crucial aspects of that testimony. The testimony in quotations is verbatim from the transcript.

On March 10, 1980, Jean S. Harris, the 56-year-old headmistress of the Madeira School for Girls, left her home in Virginia to drive, as she had many times before, to the house in the town of Harrison, Westchester County, New York, of Dr. Herman Tarnower, her 69-year-old companion and paramour for

*Previously published, under the same title, in the March/April 1985 edition of *Medical Heritage*, pp. 99–113. Reprinted with permission from W. B. Saunders Co.

Figure 4.1. Drawing of the four bullet wounds, namely, right hand, right arm, right chest above the clavicle, and right posterior shoulder. The prosecution contended initially that there were four separate bullets causing the four wounds and later that three separate bullets caused them. The defense claimed that the four wounds were caused by four separate bullets.

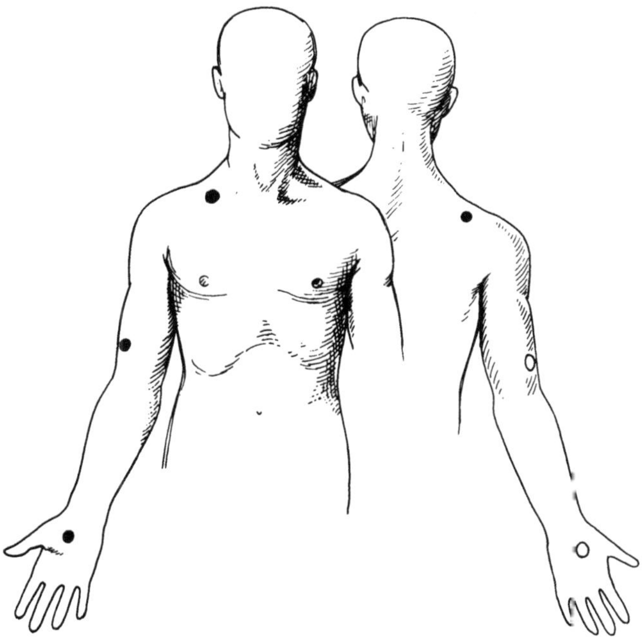

the past 14 years. This time she carried a suicide note and a .32 caliber revolver in her pocketbook. She arrived at Tarnower's home at about 10:45 P.M. By 10:55 P.M., Tarnower was mortally wounded, with bullet wounds in the right side of his chest, and right shoulder, arm, and hand. When she was arrested, Mrs. Harris was noted by police and correction officers to have bruises on her left arm and on the left side of her upper lip. Blood was later identified on her brassiere by a serologist. The defense claimed that the shooting was a "tragic accident" and that the doctor had been shot during a struggle as he attempted to prevent Mrs. Harris from committing suicide. The prosecution claimed that Mrs. Harris shot the doctor in a "jealous rage" because he had jilted her in favor of a younger woman, his 38-year-old office assistant. On February 24, 1981, Mrs. Harris was convicted of murder and on March 20, 1981, she was sentenced to from 15 years to life in prison.

On December 30, 1981, in rejecting the bid of Jean Harris for a new trial in the murder of Dr. Herman Tarnower, Presiding Justice Milton Mollen of the Appellate Division, Second Department, of the Supreme Court of the State of

New York, wrote that, although Mrs. Harris "did not receive a perfect trial, she received an eminently fair one." But if the trial was fair by legal standards, was it also fair by medical ones?

Some sense of the importance of the role of "expert" testimony about cutaneous histology in the trial of Jean Harris may be gathered from the written opinion of Justice Mollen on appeal:

> An extraordinary amount of expert testimony was offered at trial on a variety of subjects. The major dispute turned out to be whether the bullet which entered and exited Dr. Tarnower's hand went on to cause his chest wound. The People contended that it did and that that fact would suggest that the injury to Tarnower's hand was a 'defensive wound.' The defense argued that the hand and chest wounds had been caused by two separate bullets. Opinions were offered in support of the prosecution's theory, and in contradiction to it, largely depending upon whether the particular expert was able to discern in the slides of the chest wound evidence of cells which were peculiar to the palmar surface of the hand.

During the trial of Mrs. Harris, which began on November 21, 1980, and ended on February 24, 1981, six general pathologists and two dermatopathologists were called to the stand by the defense and by the prosecutor to testify about matters pertaining to histology of the skin. The meaning of those issues in the trial of Jean Harris may be best understood if crucial events and opinions are presented in chronological sequence. Readers may now serve as peer reviewers.

CHRONOLOGY OF EVENTS RELATING TO THE TESTIMONY OF PATHOLOGISTS

March 10, 1980—Dr. Herman Tarnower dies of bullet wounds. Jean Harris is arrested and charged with murder in the second degree.

March 11, 1980—An autopsy is performed by Drs. Louis Roh, deputy medical examiner, and Gary Paparo, chief medical examiner of Westchester County. Dr. Roh's autopsy report describes four bullet wounds and tells of four separate bullets entering the body of Dr. Tarnower.

March 14, 1980—Preliminary hearing. Dr. Roh testifies that four separate bullets had entered the body of Dr. Tarnower.

March 21, 1980—Dr. Roh issues an autopsy report titled "Histologic Examination" and in the wound in the chest notes only ". . . fresh hemorrhage in subcutaneous tissue and adipose tissue. Dermis shows coagulation necrosis of collagen fibers. A few foci of gun powder deposit are seen in subcutaneous tissue."

March 24, 1980—Grand jury. Roh testifies that the wound in the hand is consistent with an attempt to defend against a gun being fired and that the victim's wounds are not consistent with a struggle. He again states that four separate bullets entered the body of Dr. Tarnower, but that only three of them were recovered from the body. No bullet was recovered from the hand wound because it was an "in and out, through and through" wound. The fourth bullet was never found.

November 21, 1980—Trial of *The People v. Jean S. Harris* begins at Westchester County Court House, Judge Russell R. Leggett presiding.

December 18, 1980—Dr. Roh is called to the stand by the prosecutor, George Bolen, assistant district attorney for Westchester County. Dr. Roh now testifies that only three separate bullets entered the body of Dr. Tarnower. The defense was not given notice of this change of expert testimony.

January 4, 1981—During the presentation of the case for the defense, Mr. Bolen places a telephone call to Dr. Henry Ryan, chief medical examiner for the State of Maine, and learns that the doctor is in Westchester County. The same day, Mr. Thomas Lalla, assistant district attorney, visits the law office of Mr. Joel Aurnou, chief counsel for the defense, and learns that a conference is being held there among experts for the defense. Bolen later acknowledges that he surmised that Dr. Ryan was among those at the meeting in Aurnou's office. Aurnou had hired Dr. Ryan as an expert for the defense months earlier.

January 6, 1981—Mr. Bolen telephones Dr. Ryan a second time in Maine, ostensibly to respond to a Christmas card the Bolens had received from Dr. Ryan, who had been a deputy medical examiner of Westchester County. Dr. Ryan had sold his home in Westchester to Mr. Bolen before moving to Maine. On Bolen's initiative, they discuss the Harris trial. Bolen asks Dr. Ryan how one can prove that a wound in a palm is defensive, and Dr. Ryan tells him that the evidence is suggestive if specialized nerve endings (Meissner's and Vater-Pacini's) are found ectopically in the wound in the skin of the chest. Bolen calls Dr. Roh and tells him to look for pieces of palm skin (apparently not specifically for Meissner's and Pacini's corpuscles) in the histologic sections of the wound in the chest of Dr. Tarnower.

January 8, 1981—Dr. Roh writes an addendum to his histologic report of March 21, 1980, in which he claims to have found "three fragments of tissue in the bullet track in subcutaneous tissue—histologically consistent with stratum corneum, stratum lucidum, and portion of stratum granulosum of epidermis of skin." The addendum makes no specific mention of palmar skin.

January 9, 1981—Hearing on a motion for a mistrial. Aurnou asks for a mistrial on the grounds that the prosecutor had invaded the councils of the defense and violated the defendant's rights by calling an expert hired by the defense in order to learn the strategy of the defense. Bolen admits calling Ryan and discussing signs of the "defensive wound" and the importance of searching for tactile nerve endings from a palm in the wound in the skin of the chest.

Judge Leggett rules against Aurnou's motion for a mistrial. He acknowledges that Bolen had called Dr. Ryan for the specific purpose of discussing the Harris trial, but the judge holds Ryan responsible for discussing the case with Bolen.

Further, the judge holds that there is no rule that precludes a prosecutor from talking to a defendant's witness. The judge states, moreover, that he does not find that the prosecutor discussed the strategy of the defense.

Mr. Lalla tells Judge Leggett and Aurnou, in response to Aurnou's request for a single histologic slide containing the disputed fragments, that no slide may be examined "in any place other than in the office of the medical examiner," according to the "policy of the medical examiner's office." (See entries for January 15, 22, 25 and February 8, 1981.)

January 14, 1981—Dr. Paparo contacts Dr. Martin H. Brownstein, a dermatopathologist whose private laboratory is in Great Neck, Long Island, about examining the tissue sections from the chest wound of Dr. Tarnower.

January 15, 1981—Dr. Roh takes histologic slides and photomicrographs to Brownstein's office in Great Neck, Long Island.

January 16, 1981—Dr. Roh is called to the stand by Aurnou. Roh acknowledges that Bolen called him after speaking to Dr. Ryan and told him to look for skin from the palm in the skin of the chest wound. Dr. Roh testifies to finding the fragments and to writing a new report. He does not know of any nerve corpuscles specific for the skin of a palm. Roh also testifies that he did not line up the wound in the right palm with the wound in the chest at the time of the autopsy on March 10, 1980, in order to determine if they could be put into a straight alignment and, if so, in what relative positions.

Dr. Ryan is called to the stand by Aurnou and confirms the content of the telephone calls with Mr. Bolen. He disagrees with Dr. Roh about the wounds in the palm being defensive and, instead, says that they could have resulted from a struggle. He also disagrees with him about the fragments being from the epidermis of the palm. Dr. Ryan says the fragments are connective tissues; that one piece is cartilage, another consistent with joint capsule; and the third fragment he cannot identify.

Dr. Ryan disagrees with Dr. Roh about the latter's statement of lack of specificity of Meissner's and Vater-Pacini's corpuscles. Dr. Rayan says that these corpuscles are virtually specific for the skin of palms and soles.

January 19, 1981—Dr. J. N. P. Davies, Professor of Pathology at the Albany Medical School and consultant to the New York State Police Laboratory, is called to the stand by Aurnou. He disagrees with Dr. Roh about the three fragments being from the epidermis of a palm. For Dr. Davies, one piece is, undoubtedly cartilage and another piece is traumatized fibrous tissue. Davies also disagrees with Roh about the palmar wound resulting from a defensive posture rather than from a struggle.

Also that day, Dr. A. Bernard Ackerman, Professor of Dermatology and Pathology and Director of Dermatopathology at New York University Medical Center, is contacted by Aurnou and asked to examine the three fragments.

January 21, 1981—Dr. Cyril Wecht, former Coroner of Allegheny County, Pennsylvania, takes the stand for the defense. He disagrees with Dr. Roh about

Figure 4.2. (*top*). Drawing of the bullet track in the subcutaneous fat of the wound of the right chest to show the location of the three fragments in dispute. The prosecution contended that all three fragments came from epidermis of palm, whereas the defense contended that they did not. (*bottom row*). Closer views of the three fragments to illustrate that only the second fragment contains nuclei. No well-defined cell outlines can be found in the first or third fragments.

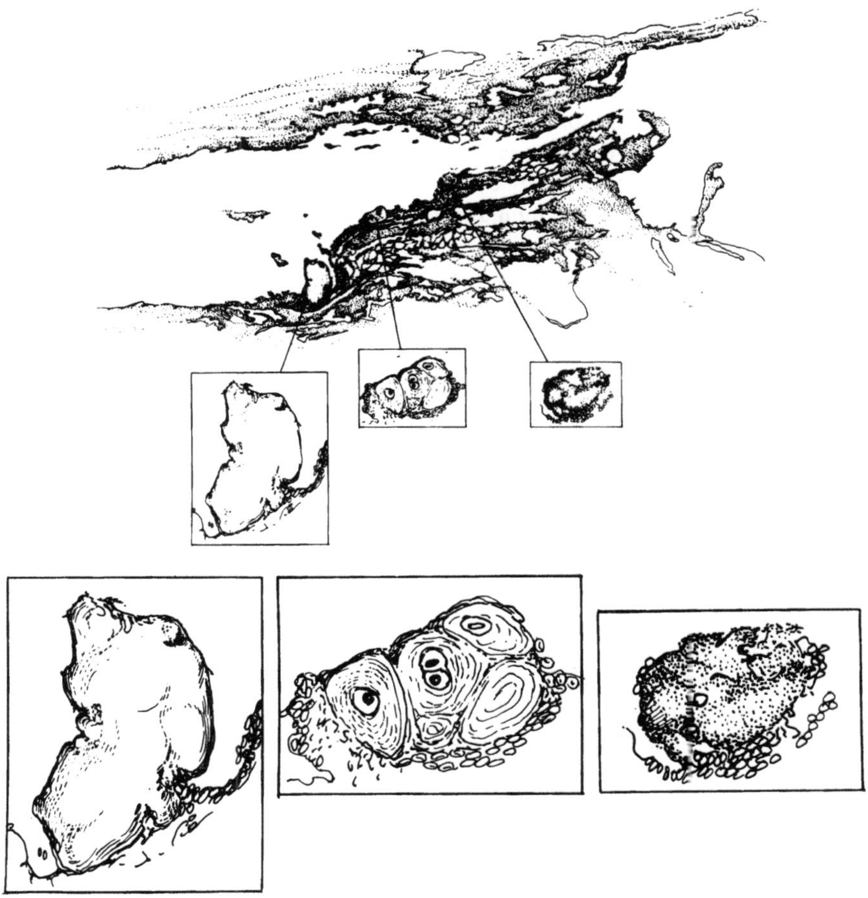

the fragments coming from a palm. He diagnoses all three fragments as connective tissue, one piece being cartilage, the other two collagen.

Also that day, Ackerman, accompanied by Victor Grossman, another attorney for the defense, goes to the medical examiner's office to review the sections of tissue from the wounds in the skin of Dr. Tarnower. For an hour Drs. Ackerman,

Roh, Paparo, and Sommers (another deputy medical examiner) discuss the fragments in question. Contrary to the opinions expressed by Dr. Roh in that wide-ranging discussion, Dr. Ackerman tells Roh, Paparo, and Sommers that: (1) there are no nuclei in the normal cornified layer and therefore the second fragment with the four nuclei cannot be from the stratum corneum; (2) granules are not present in the first and second fragments, they are present upon and around rather than within the third fragment, and the granules are finer than granules of keratohyaline, so that none of the fragments can be from the granular layer; and (3) there is no true stratum lucidum (that being an antiquated term for the lowermost portion of the stratum corneum which takes less stain). Even if there were a true stratum lucidum, no part of the tissue in any of the fragments stains less than other parts. In short, Dr. Ackerman tells Dr. Roh that all three fragments are kinds of connective tissue, probably cartilage, because the second fragment was cartilage with near certainty and the other two fragments were situated near it. The third fragment is too minute and too distorted to be identified by anyone with certainty.

January 22, 1981—Dr. Roh takes slides and photomicrographs to Dr. Brownstein's home in Great Neck. Brownstein examines them for the second time.

January 23, 1981—Dr. Ackerman is called to the stand by Mr. Aurnou. Using a blackboard, he draws diagrams of epidermis from palm and chest skin and explains that the three fragments do not consist of epidermis from the palm, but, because the second fragment is almost certainly cartilage, all three of the closely situated fragments are probably cartilage.

On cross examination, Mr. Bolen raises, for the first time, the possibility that the second fragment with the four nuclei is from the spinous layer of the skin of a palm of Dr. Tarnower. Ackerman rejects that possibility on the ground that a fragment that size from the spinous layer should have many more nuclei, not merely four.

Also on January 23, Mr. Aurnou calls Drs. Alfred Angrist, professor and chairman emeritus of the Department of Pathology at Albert Einstein College of Medicine, and Michel Janis, professor of Pathology at Albert Einstein College of Medicine, to the stand. Both disagree with Dr. Roh that the three fragments consist of epidermis from a palm. Angrist considers the fragments to be cartilage or altered collagen. Janis interprets some of the fragments to be fibrocartilage and insists that none are keratin.

Bolen: Is it possible that any of these three fragments could be keratin?

Janis: Is it possible that any of these three fragments could be keratin? No, it's not possible.

Bolen: It's not possible at all?

Janis: It's not possible at all.

January 25, 1981—Dr. Roh, Mr. Bolen, and Mr. Lalla take the slides and photomicrographs to Dr. Brownstein's home in Great Neck, where Brownstein examines them for the third time.

Figure 4.3. Drawing of epidermis of normal skin of the plam (*left*) and of the chest (*right*) to illustrate the contrast between the compactly arranged cornified cells in a thick cornified layer of the palm and the basket-weave arrangement of cornified cells in the thin cornified layer of the skin of the chest and the contrast between the thick granular layer of epidermis of palm and the thin granular layer of epidermis of chest. The epidermis of palm and chest, like that of the entire integument, consists of four layers, namely, basal, spinous, granular and cornified.

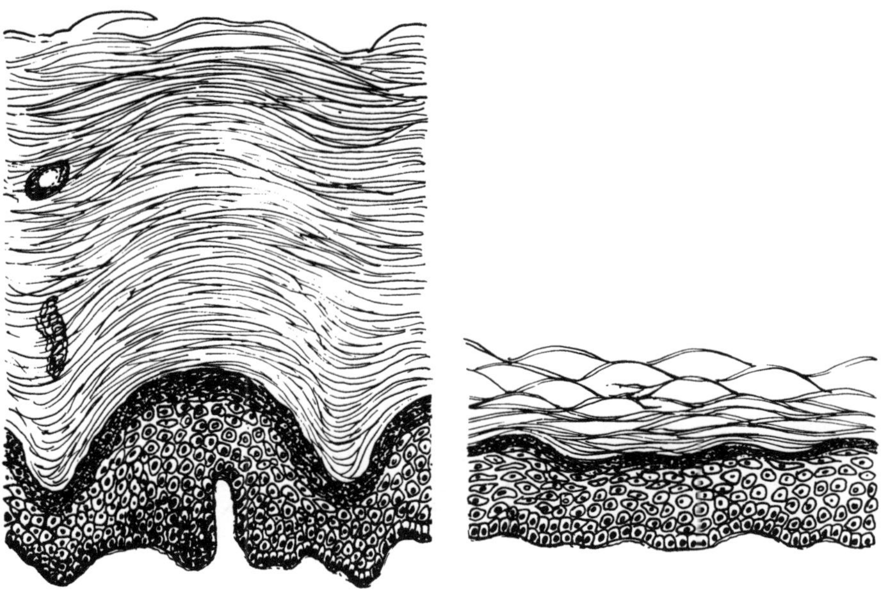

February 4, 1981—Dr. Brownstein writes a report about his findings in the wound of the skin of the chest. He notes small fragments in the subcutaneous tissue, but describes only one of them and concludes on the basis of that one fragment that "there is material in the chest wound that is quite consistent with the type of keratin found on palms and soles." He gives no interpretation for the other two fragments.

February 8, 1981—Messrs. Bolen and Lalla again take slides and photomicrographs to Brownstein's home in Great Neck. Brownstein examines them for the fourth time.

February 10, 1981—Dr. Ackerman, at the request of Aurnou, sits at the counsel table in the courtroom to assist counsel and does that for the duration of the trial.

Dr. Roh returns to the stand for the third time, this time called by Bolen. Roh again states that the palmar wound was sustained by Dr. Tarnower in self-defense and that fragments from the palm were carried by the bullet into the wound in the skin of the chest.

Figure 4.4. Drawing of cornified, granular, and spinous cells in the epidermis. Dr. Roh contended that the three fragments consisted of various combinations of these cells (and cells of the "stratum lucidum"). Note the intercellular spines between the spinous cells, a sine qua non for identification of spinous cells by conventional microscopy. Dr. Roh eventually testified that the second fragment consisted of spinous cells, but he acknowledged that no intercellular spines were identifiable in that fragment.

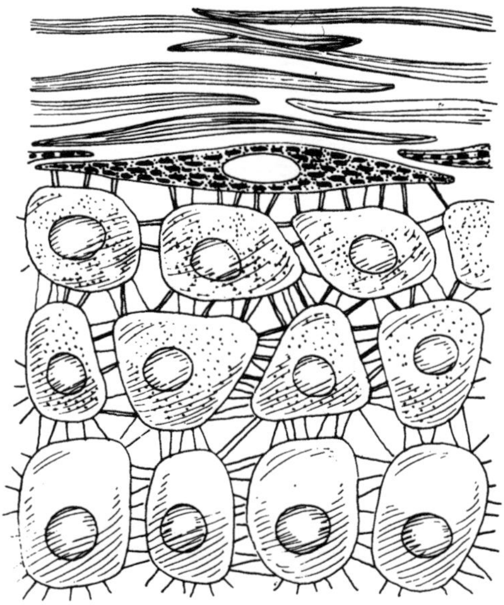

Roh projects 23 photomicrographs of skin tissue from the wounds in the palm and chest of Dr. Tarnower and explains his interpretations to the jury. Roh testifies that the largest fragment is from the keratin layer of the palm, the second fragment with the nuclei from the spinous layer of the palm, and the third and smallest fragment from the granular layer of the palm.

February 11, 1981—Dr. Roh is cross-examined by Aurnou. He tells Aurnou that the largest fragment is stratum corneum, the second fragment stratum spinosum close to the granular layer, and the third fragment stratum lucidum close to the granular layer.

Dr. Roh acknowledges to Aurnou that he had left the spinous layer out of his addendum of January 8, 1981, and insists to Aurnou that collagen is a cell with a nucleus, cytoplasm, and cell membrane. He also insists that there are no nuclei in the cells of the granular layer of the epidermis. Aurnou questions Roh about the same 23 photomicrographs that were projected the previous day. Many inconsistencies emerge.

Dr. Roh is inconsistent about whether he had had any discussion with Ackerman in the medical examiner's office on January 21, 1981. Aurnou asks him "did there occur a dialogue between you and Dr. Ackerman?" and Roh replies

Figure 4.5. The histologic differentiation of epithelial from connective tissue is apparent in this drawing of epidermis and dermis. The epidermis shows all of the features of epithelium, whereas the dermis shows those of connective tissue.

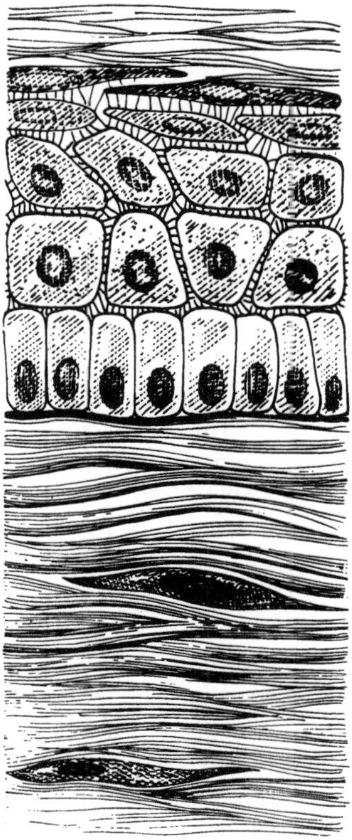

"Yes," but shortly thereafter Roh tells Aurnou that, "I didn't say a word . . . I just listened."

February 12, 1981—Dr. Brownstein is called to the stand by Bolen. Having only commented about one of the fragments in his written report, Brownstein now testifies that two of the fragments are quite consistent with the type of tissue found in the outer layer of the skin of palms and soles. He is not certain of the second fragment with the four nuclei.

Dr. Brownstein disagrees with Dr. Roh on 23 separate issues of fact concerning the three fragments in particular and cutaneous histology in general. Dr. Brownstein admits that he wrote a note in his own hand, presumably to Mr. Bolen, suggesting that good photographic evidence will frighten off the possibility of other dermatopathologists testifying in the case.

Dr. Ackerman is called back to the stand by Aurnou. He disagrees with the testimony of Drs. Roh and Brownstein that the fragments come from epidermis of a palm and reiterates that they consist of connective tissue, probably cartilage.

The defense and the prosecution rest their cases.

February 16, 1981—Summations by Aurnou and Bolen. Aurnou spends much of his summation on the physical evidence and especially on the matters of cutaneous histology. Bolen spends little time on the physical evidence and on the cutaneous histology.

February 17, 1981—Judge Leggett charges the jury. He reviews the testimony of every one of the eight pathologists who testified during the trial. His emphasis to the jury is on the question of intent, i.e., did Mrs. Harris intend to kill Herman Tarnower or did she not. The three fragments in dispute are relevant to the question of intent.

February 24, 1981—After eight days, the jury announced its verdict: Guilty, on all counts. Mrs. Harris is imprisoned in the Westchester County Jail.

March 20, 1981—Judge Leggett sentences Mrs. Harris to 15 years in prison. The prisoner is taken to the Bedford Hills Correctional Center in Westchester County, New York.

December 30, 1981—Mrs. Harris' appeal is denied in a unanimous decision by the Appellate Division of the Supreme Court of the State of New York.

November 16, 1982—Mrs. Harris' appeal is denied in a unanimous decision by the New York State Court of Appeals.

March 21, 1983—The United States Supreme Court declines to review the decision of the New York State Court of Appeals.

These excerpts from the transcripts of the trial in point compel us, in my view, to confront this question: Did the testimony and practices of the expert medical witnesses serve the interests of a fair trial by assuring that the jury, who as lay people necessarily rely on the expertness of medical witnesses, was presented with accurate statements of facts for their deliberation and determination of guilt or innocence? To illustrate the gravity of that question, the following progression of facts is highlighted:

1. That by changing his testimony about the number of separate bullets that entered the body of Herman Tarnower from four to three, Dr. Roh created the issue of a "defensive wound." In his autopsy report of March 11, 1980, at the preliminary hearing on March 14, 1980, and before the Grand Jury on March 24, 1980, Dr. Roh stated that four separate bullets had entered the body of the late Dr. Tarnower. On December 18, 1980, during the trial, Dr. Roh changed his testimony from four bullets to three. This change of testimony raised the notion of a "defensive wound," suggesting intent on the part of Mrs. Harris, and created the prosecution's theory of a "defensive wound" rather than a wound suffered during a struggle.

2. That during the trial on January 6 and 7, 1981, during the presentation of the case for the defense, the prosecutor, Mr. Bolen, telephoned Dr. Henry Ryan, whom he knew to be an expert witness for the defense, and initiated a discussion of the case. Bolen asked Ryan during at least one conversation how one could prove that a bullet had been fired with intent to kill and, in particular, the bullet(s) that went through the right hand and chest of Dr. Tarnower. Ryan advised Bolen

that finding specialized nerves from palmar skin in the wound in the skin of the chest would indicate that the late doctor's right palm had been held up in a posture of self-defense.

If Mr. Bolen did not consider his conversations with Dr. Ryan to be improper or unfair, why, during his interrogation by Aurnou and Lalla in the Mistrial Hearing before Judge Leggett on January 19, 1981, did he attempt to explain his calls to Ryan as being little more than social and belated Christmas greetings. Bolen: "What I am saying to you is this, Mr. Aurnou. When I called Dr. Ryan at his home in Maine—and I did that in consultation with my wife with respect to a card we had received . . . " Judge Leggett, in his ruling against a mistrial, stated that "On the motion for a mistrial and the hearing that followed, I make the following findings of fact. I find that the district attorney called a person known to him, Dr. Ryan, and there being an acquaintanceship, that might not rise to friendship, but certainly it was more than a casual meeting, and I would also find that the prosecutor under the circumstances presented in the hearing obviously called, in my opinion, to discuss the case after having discussed the niceties of it insofar as to sound out the doctor in certain aspects of it . . . I find that the facts indicate that the prosecutor did bring the conversation around to the Harris matter to the extent that he discussed with Dr. Roh certainly the theory of it, the defensive wound in general; and Dr. Ryan also discussed other cases of what might be described as defensive wounds, and when I use that term I am indicating that the doctor told Mr. Bolen that there were certain methods of determining the, let's call it the transference of tissue from one area of the body being carried by a moving bullet—and bringing it to another area.

"I would also find that Mr. Bolen brought up the question about the possibility of a bullet going through a hand and into a chest; and again discussing this defensive wound—and I use that only insofar as it describes a hand wound in relation to the shoulder in the context in which Mr. Bolen has presented it and in which the testimony was elicited—the doctor indicated there was only one definitive way to show that one bullet had made the two wounds in a hand and a chest, and that was to look for palmar tissue, if that is the term, in the chest cavity to see whether residuals were there."

3. That in the midst of the trial Dr. Roh, after a telephone call from Mr. Bolen, changed his findings about the wound in the chest and that his new findings lent support to the prosecution contention of a wound sustained in self-defense. Following the telephone call and instructions from Bolen, Dr. Roh reviewed the histologic sections of skin from the chest wound. Two days after Bolen's telephone conversations with Dr. Ryan and then with himself, Roh wrote an addendum to his original histologic report of March 21, 1980. In the original histologic report, Dr. Roh did not mention any fragments from palmar skin in the skin of the chest wound. In his addendum, Roh wrote that in the bullet track in the subcutaneous tissue there were three tiny fragments of tissue histologically consistent with stratum corneum, stratum lucidum, and stratum granulosum of epidermis of skin, presumably of the palm. He also asserted in that addendum

that there was gunpowder near one of the fragments. This supported the prosecution's contention of a wound sustained in self-defense rather than a struggle.

4. That Bolen introduced the issue of the second fragment consisting of cells from the spinous layer when that layer of epidermis was never mentioned in Dr. Roh's addendum. Bolen asked Dr. Ackerman during cross-examination on January 23, 1981 whether the second fragment with the four nuclei could be from the spinous layer, though Dr. Roh's addendum never mentioned the spinous layer at all. Bolen introduced the spinous layer of the epidermis as an explanation for the second fragment, presumably because Dr. Roh had learned from his discussion with Dr. Ackerman in the Medical Examiner's office on January 21, 1981 that the normal stratum corneum (including the "stratum lucidum") does not contain nuclei; yet his addendum to the autopsy report had implied that the second fragment with the four nuclei consisted of stratum corneum. Dr. Roh testified incorrectly in court that granular cells in the granular layer do not contain nuclei, so that for him the second fragment with the four nuclei could not possibly consist of granular cells. Furthermore, that second fragment did not contain any granules. On February 10, 1981, Dr. Roh, under direct examination by Bolen, stated that the second fragment consisted of spinous layer of epidermis from a palm, and repeated his assertion to Aurnou on cross-examination on February 11, 1981. These changes in Roh's testimony lent validity to the prosecution claim that the wounds in the palm and the chest resulted from a single bullet fired with intent by Mrs. Harris.

5. That the policy of the medical examiner's office did not apply equally to the defense and to the prosecution. In the mistrial hearing on January 9, 1981, Aurnou asked Judge Leggett for a single histologic slide from the medical examiner's office that showed the disputed fragments in order that pathologists for the defense might examine the histologic sections at their own microscopes and not have to journey to the medical examiner's office in Westchester. Mr. Thomas Lalla, assistant district attorney, told Judge Leggett that "I just want the court to be aware of the fact that there is a policy of the medical examiner's office not to release these slides to anyone other than their own personnel and *not to have them examined in any place other than in the office of the medical examiner*[my italics], so they may want to be heard on this specific issue." On January 15, 22, and 25, 1981, and on February 8, 1981, the histologic slides were taken from the medical examiner's office to the office (once) and the home (thrice) of Dr. Martin H. Brownstein, a dermatopathologist who had been hired by the prosecution. On January 25 and on February 8, it was Mr. Lalla (in the company of Dr. Roh and Mr. Bolen on January 25 and with Mr. Bolen alone on February 8) who took the slides to Dr. Brownstein's home, contrary to the stated policy of the medical examiner's office that he had articulated to Judge Leggett.

6. That Dr. Brownstein gave testimony about the fragments in court that differed from his written report. On February 4, 1981, after having examined the histologic sections containing the fragments on four separate occasions, to say nothing of reviewing hundreds of photomicrographs of them, Dr. Brownstein

wrote a report that addressed itself to only one of the three fragments. Of this fragment he wrote that it "is quite consistent with the type of keratin found on palms and soles." But Dr. Brownstein wrote nothing about the identity of the other two fragments, which he had studied on four separate occasions and which had been the object of attention of seven other pathologists. During direct examination by Bolen on February 12, 1981, Dr. Brownstein testified that two of the three fragments were consistent with the stratum corneum from the palm of the late doctor. But Dr. Brownstein told Aurnou on cross-examination that he "could not identify" the second fragment with the four nuclei "with any certainty." Brownstein admitted to Aurnou that he believed that the three fragments were all of one tissue ("I would like to think that all three [fragments] came from the same piece of tissue"), implying the stratum corneum, but the second fragment had four nuclei so it could not possibly be from stratum corneum. Dr. Roh accounted for the four nuclei in the second fragment by changing his testimony about that fragment from stratum corneum to stratum spinosum. Dr. Brownstein simply stated that he could not identify the second fragment, despite the fact that it was considerably larger and better preserved than the third fragment, which he said he could identify as stratum corneum.

7. That Dr. Brownstein recommended strategy to "frighten off possibility" of other dermapathologists testifying. In notes presumably for Mr. Bolen, written in Brownstein's own hand and given by the prosecutor to the attorney for the defense, Brownstein wrote that "good photog evidence will frighten off possibility of other dermatopath testify."

Aurnou: Now, you mentioned that you had come here to help us in a search for the truth; is that correct?

Brownstein: That is quite correct.

Aurnou: Did you ever consider yourself to be an advocate for either side?

Brownstein: No.

Aurnou: You would have had no interest, for example, in discouraging the testimony of any other doctor who might, for example, disagree with you?

Brownstein: No way.

Aurnou: And did you prepare certain notes, in connection with this case?

Brownstein: Yes, I did.

Aurnou: And in your notes, Doctor, did you make the statement in your own handwriting that good photographic evidence will frighten off the possibility of other dermatopathologists who testify?

Brownstein: If it is in the notes I probably did write that.

Aurnou: In a search for truth, Doctor, or as another advocate? Come on, Doctor, give us an answer.

Brownstein: I was preparing my position and . . .

Aurnou: And you hoped to scare off other competent physicians. *That* is in a search for the truth?

Why did Dr. Brownstein want to "frighten off" other dermatopathologists from testifying in a judicial procedure convened for the purpose of determining the truth? Should a defendant not be permitted, even encouraged, in the spirit of truth and fairness, to have other dermatopathologists examine those same fragments and offer their opinions about them?

8. That critical parts of Dr. Roh's testimony concerning cutaneous histology were, in my opinion, inaccurate. The fragments of tissue in the wound of the chest identified as palmar epidermis by Drs. Roh and Brownstein were offered by the prosecution to suggest that Mrs. Harris had shot Dr. Tarnower with the intention of killing him. Whether these minuscule fragments, the largest 0.2 mm × 0.1 mm according to Brownstein's own measurement, were epithelial, as claimed by Roh and Brownstein, or connective tissue, as contended by the six pathologists who testified for the defense, was crucial to the defense of Mrs. Harris. (See *Chronology* above.)

This is what Dr. Roh had to say about collagen, the major connective tissue in the body, when he was cross-examined:

Aurnou: This is your report of March 21, 1980. First of all, you said you found in the dermis of the right chest coagulation necrosis of collagen fibers. Have I quoted you correctly, Doctor?

Roh: Correct.

Aurnou: What is necrosis?

Roh: Necrosis means simply the death of a cell.

Aurnou: Death?

Roh: Yes.

Aurnou: Is collagen alive?

Roh: Collagen—

Aurnou: Was it ever alive?

Mr. Bolen: He was about to answer a question and he went on to the next.

The Court: I will take the two questions and consider them as one. The way they were framed, they are the same. You can either break it down or you can have it reframed, if you want.

Roh: Collagen is a cell. If a human being is made out of a cell, if the human being is alive, the collagen cell is alive.

Aurnou: Isn't it a fact that collagen is not a cell at all, Doctor?

Roh: What is it, then?

Aurnou: How about a fiber?

Roh: A fiber is a cell.

Aurnou: Doctor, what is a fibroblast?

Roh: That's a cell, too.

Aurnou: What does a fibroblast do with regard to collagen?

Roh: Fibroblast is considered as a precursor of the immatured form of the collagen.

Aurnou: Isn't a fibroblast the cell that makes, spins out, collagen?

Roh: Fibroblast becomes collagen fibers.

Aurnou: Doctor, does collagen have a nucleus, in your opinion?

Roh: Collagen fibers, yes.

Aurnou: What does that consist of, Doctor?

Roh: Nucleus?

Aurnou: No, Doctor. The particular nucleus of a collagen, as you call it, cell, . . . Can you describe for the jury [as] consistent with accepted medical literature?

Roh: Of collagen fibers?

Aurnou: Collagen cell, Doctor. You used that term didn't you?

Roh: Collagen fiber is a collagen cell. It's made of cells. It has a nucleus in it.

Aurnou: I am going to try again, Doctor. Isn't it a fact (A) that collagen is a fiber and (B) that it has no nucleus at all?

Roh: Yes, they do.

Aurnou: Now, in all fairness, Doctor, I will ask the question over. Is collagen not the major extracellular component of the—

Roh: Cell.

Aurnou: Of the body. Extracellular, Doctor. Do you understand that means outside the cell, Doctor?

Roh: Yes. I would say it's the extracellular portion of the cell.

Aurnou: Doctor, isn't that a non sequitur? In other words, a thing is either a cell or part of a cell or outside a cell.

Roh: Anything in the human body is part of the cell.

Aurnou: Part of the body, Doctor, not part of the cell.

Roh: The human body is made of cells.

Aurnou: Are you telling me, then, Doctor, as you understand medicine, as you understand pathology, as you understand histology, that there is no extracellular protein in the body?

Roh: Yes, there is. It is part of the cell.

Aurnou at last asked Roh: Doctor, would you agree or disagree with this sentence: Examination of collagen in connective tissues by light microscopy demonstrates that collagen is deposited as large bundles of regularly-oriented fibers which on further examination can be shown to be composed of fibrils and microfibrils?

Roh: Yes.

Aurnou: Doctor, do you know what the criteria are histologically or morphologically for identifying collagen fibers?

Roh: That's exactly what you read.

How could Roh exclude the possibility that the three fragments in the wound in the skin of the chest of Dr. Tarnower consisted of connective tissue if he has faulty criteria for recognizing collagen under the microscope?

9. That, in my judgment, Dr. Brownstein did not on his own present accurately the morphologic criteria for differentiating epithelial from connective tissue, the criteria upon which the matter of the three fragments turned. This is what Dr. Brownstein had to say about differentiating epithelial from connective tissue when he was cross-examined:

Arnou: Well, perhaps you would be kind enough to give us the criteria, for example, Doctor, that differentiate cells of that [epithelial] layer from the connective tissue.

Brownstein: Oh, yes. In terms of looking under the microscope and looking at cells, for example, if you wanted to decide about a certain fragment, decide whether they come from the outer layers of the skin, the epidermis, or whether they come from the deeper tissues like the connective tissue, collagen or cartilage, there are certain criteria to distinguish them. If we are talking about the outermost layer of the skin, the epidermis, does not have nuclei, this is one of the factors differentiating epidermis from cells like cartilage cells or keratin cells which could have nuclei.

Aurnou: Well, doctor, let's go back to my question about the differentiation [of epithelial from connective tissue]. This is the question we all got sidetracked on and I will repeat it for you, sir. Differentiation between epithelial tissue and connective tissue, and I am particularly concerned that you be kind enough to give the jury the criteria for that distinction.

Brownstein: Okay. I would say a very important one is that if we see cells, the cells in the epidermis tend to be more oval-shaped, where cells from collagen for example, might tend to be very flat and very elongated, sort of spindle-shaped.

Aurnou: Any others?

Brownstein: Any other criteria for differentiating epithelial cells from—

Aurnou: Epithelial cells from the connective tissue cells.

Brownstein: This is one of the main criteria.

Aurnou: May I offer you some, Doctor.

Brownstein: Yes.

Aurnou: Is it not correct that in epithelium, the cells are cohesive, the first thing you could observe about them is that they touch one another?

Brownstein: Yes.

Aurnou: Back in the spinous layer you actually find intercellular bridges between one cell and another?

Brownstein: Yes.

Aurnou: Now the next thing I would like to ask you is whether or not this question of shape you spoke about is not one which is confusing and misleading because in particular, fibroblasts which are found in connective tissue are often oval-shaped, Doctor?

Brownstein: Yes, it is possible. We are talking in simplifications now.

Aurnou: I understand that, but what I am trying to get you to do, as you said, use language that will have meaning to the ladies and gentlemen of the jury.

Brownstein: Okay.

Aurnou: So oval-shaped can be oval-shaped cells in the stratum corneum or it can also be fibroblasts?

Brownstein: Yes.

Aurnou: Now, Doctor, let's return to the differentiation between epithelial and connective tissue. You have told us that you agree with my suggestion that the cells of the epithelial layer are cohesive, and they touch one another and we would readily expect to see that happen?

Brownstein: Yes.

Aurnou: Is that true of connective tissue, Doctor?

Brownstein: Generally not.

Aurnou: Would it also be fair for me to say that the cells of epithelial tissue—of connective tissue, I'm sorry, are not cohesive?

Brownstein: Generally true, yes.

The Court: I did not hear the end of the question, I'm sorry.

Mr. Aurnou: Are not cohesive, Your Honor.

Aurnou: Would it also be fair for me to suggest to you, Doctor, that the cells from connective tissue are scattered amidst anuclear extracellular material?

Brownstein: That is generally true.

Aurnou: And there is quite a distance, sometimes, between the cells in connective tissue; correct?

Brownstein: Correct.

Aurnou: Now, I would like to turn for just a moment to collagen, which, we can agree, is one of the connective tissues; correct?

Brownstein: Yes.

Aurnou: Is it a living cell?

Brownstein: Yes.

Aurnou: Collagen is a living cell?

Brownstein: Collagen is not a cell, no. It is a material that is secreted by a cell.

10. That Dr. Roh stated about a fragment of tissue only micra in diameter: "The major portion of the smallest fragment is lucidum layer, but since there is a transition between the granular layer to the lucidum layer, a small portion of granule was attached to the particular section, the fragment." In my opinion, no human being can make such a determination on a fragment of tissue that minute.

11. That Dr. Roh projected photomicrographs to the jury that he and Dr. Brownstein acknowledged were out of focus when the purpose of the photo-

micrographs was to convince the jury that three minuscule fragments consisted of "stratum corneum, stratum lucidum, and stratum granulosum."

Aurnou: And finally, are any of the photomicrographs out of focus, Doctor?

Roh: Well, I am not a professional photographer. So some of them are out of focus.

Aurnou: Tell us about the quality of these photomicrographs, Doctor?

Brownstein: The quality was quite satisfactory to make the points, but I would have done things a little differently.

Aurnou: Well, for one thing, Doctor, would you tell me please if in these photomicrographs you found, among other things, photomicrographs that were out of focus?

Brownstein: This is not unusual. Of course, there were areas out of focus.

Aurnou: I am talking about whole photomicrographs.

Brownstein: This happens all the time. This is perfectly acceptable.

12. That the histologic sections containing the three fragments were flawed by many technical imperfections:

Aurnou: Now, with regard to the 20 to 22 [histologic slides] that you saw, Doctor, was there good contrast between the eosinophilic and the basophilic?

Brownstein: Satisfactory, but not perfect.

Aurnou: Was there good contrast?

Brownstein: Good is a relative term. I could answer that 'yes'.

Aurnou: And were there overlays?

Brownstein: Yes, there were overlays.

Aurnou: Were there tears?

Brownstein: Yes.

Aurnou: Were there knife marks?

Brownstein: I think there were knife marks, yes.

Aurnou: Was there dirt?

Brownstein: Yes.

Aurnou: Other artifacts?

Brownstein: Yes.

Aurnou: Folds?

Brownstein: Probably.

Aurnou: Aren't each one of the things that I have listed defects in the slide?

Brownstein: It is a defect in minor points of perfection, but we are not talking about perfection here. They still show the evidence with the dirt or with the tears or with anything else.

Aurnou: Doctor, wouldn't it be helpful in a matter of this importance to have slides . . .

Brownstein: They were decent. We are talking about esthetics now rather than essence.

Aurnou: I am not talking about simply out of focus photomicrographs, I am talking about the original slides which you understand have knife marks on them, tears, artifacts shown clearly, overlays, and so forth.

Brownstein: Yes.

Aurnou: Those defects obscure the diagnosis and that is what quality control is all about; is it not, Doctor?

Brownstein: Quality control tries to get satisfactory tissue sections, but these were quite satisfactory for the purpose. They weren't ideal, but they show the entire picture.

The difficulties that the technical defects posed for diagnosis of the fragments was communicated to Bolen by Dr. Angrist in this exchange:

Bolen: What did you determine those fragments to be, sir?

Angrist: Well, I can't tell you that I knew exactly what they are, but I know what they are not. They are not ordinary tissue of the palm that I can recognize. At least I cannot recognize them as such. I guess that would be a more appropriate way of putting it.

Bolen: So you can't recognize them as being tissue, let's say from the palmar surface. Is that correct?

Angrist: Correct.

Bolen: Is it possible they could have been, though?

Angrist: Anything is possible. But I doubt it.

Bolen: Well, what do you think those three fragments were, based upon your years of experience in this area? What do you think they are?

Angrist: They are debris. Some of them are dirt. There is a lot of dirt on that slide. But other than that, there were some that were altered tissues with changes in it . . .

Bolen: Did you think any of those tissues might have been cartilage?

Angrist: Some of them did mimic cartilage, yes.

Dr. Roh had denied that there were any defects in the histologic sections that his laboratory had prepared.

Aurnou: Doctor, is there overlay on this slide?

Roh: Yes.

Aurnou: Is that a defect?

Roh: It's not a defect. It's the overlay. Defect means absence of something.

Aurnou questioned Roh further.

Aurnou: Is it a defect in preparation, Doctor?

Roh: I don't think it's a very good way of doing it, but you cannot avoid it.

Aurnou: You cannot avoid it?

Roh: It does happen.

13. That Dr. Roh changed his opinion about the findings in the wound in the chest of Dr. Tarnower time after time:

March 21, 1980—Autopsy report. No palmar fragments in the wound in the skin of the chest, only "large amount of fresh hemorrhage" and "coagulation necrosis of collagen fibers."

Jan. 8, 1981—Addendum to the autopsy report. There were "three fragments of tissue in the bullet track in subcutaneous tissue of the chest wound" and "these tiny fragments are . . . histologically consistent with stratum corneum, stratum lucidum, and portion of stratum granulosum of epidermis of skin."

Jan. 16, 1981—In court. "I found a small fragment, tiny fragments of palm tissue in the deep . . . in the skin section taken from the chest." The tissues consistent with palmar skin are "the top three layers of five layers normally present in epidermis."

Feb. 10, 1981—In court. "The largest fragment I found in the chest section is similar or consistent with the histological characteristics with the keratin layer found in the palmar surface. As far as the second fragment is concerned, with the nuclei, it is consistent with the layer found on the upper part of the prickle cell layer, or spinosum layer . . . and the smallest fragment with the fine granules is consistent with the one found in the granule [sic] layer of the palm of the hand.

Feb. 11, 1981—In court.

Aurnou: Doctor, just so we are perfectly clear, I am going to refer to the largest fragment as No. 1. What portion of the skin tissue do you finally determine, in your opinion, that was?

Roh: The largest fragment, I determined that was a stratum corneum.

Aurnou: And the second fragment, the one with the nuclei, that was?

Roh: Upper layer of stratum spinosum close to the granular layer.

Aurnou: And the third and smallest.

Roh: Stratum lucidum, close to the granular layer.

The role cutaneous histology played in this trial raises many questions in addition to those of scientific accuracy, issues that are pertinent to the relationship between medicine and the law in America. For example,

Should the standards for an 'expert' in medicine be redefined?

Should physicians be brought to court as advocates for the prosecution or advocates for the defense, or should physicians be placed at the disposal of the court as advocates of truth?

In the present adversary system of justice, which embroils physicians, should there be a code of ethics that governs the behavior of physicians within that system?

What standards should govern the testimony of forensic and general pathologists in court and should there be penalties for serious violation of those standards?

Is it proper for medical examiners and prosecutors to work together as collaborating colleagues, rather than as independent professionals?

Do fees paid to physicians by defense lawyers or prosecutors tend to compromise the intellectual integrity of physicians?

Can juries of laymen understand evidence in trials in which subtle knowledge of medicine is required?

Should medical students and residents be given formal training in preparation for their possible roles in medical-legal matters?

Should the same standards of peer review that apply in medicine in general be applicable to medical testimony?

Peer review has come to be a means of maintaining high standards in the practice of medicine. In anatomic pathology, for example, histologic sections prepared in a particular laboratory and interpreted by an affiliated pathologist are often requested for review by a pathologist not of that laboratory. And if, in further example, the first pathologist had interpreted a neoplasm as benign and the neoplasm subsequently metastasized, almost always that pathologist is informed of his error by the colleague in pathology who reviewed the original and subsequent sections or by colleagues in clinical medicine or surgery who cared for the patient. The findings from laboratories of clinical pathology are scrutinized by physicians and surgeons who have to manage patients from whom specimens were submitted, and those findings must at once be judged to be in accord with clinical observations and, later, with biologic course. In short, there is a monitor, a kind of cross-check like cross-examination, built into the practice of pathology in the form of peer review and eventual or ultimate outcome. Even in the realm of the textbook literature of pathology and in journals of pathology, textual material and articles are subjected to review before and after publication by able colleagues. Thus, a pathologist's performance is not carried out in an unassailable ivory tower, but before a forum of critical colleagues and the wider community of general and specialized physicians.

A notable exception to ready review of the performance of pathologists and physicians in general occurs in courts of law. Rarely is the actual testimony of a physician in court made known to the community of physicians at large and even when a physician openly testifies in a case, he may not even look over the transcript of his own testimony, let alone that of other physicians who may also have testified in that case. This special province, the courtroom, shelters testifying physicians from corrective peer review that is so critically important to maintaining high standards in pathology and any other discipline of medicine.

Most physicians are fully cognizant of the Hippocratic standards of practice of medicine that obtain equally in a university, a hospital, and a private office.

But few physicians, I dare say, are fully aware of the deviation from those standards that all too often occurs in the courtroom. The purpose of this essay is to alert colleagues to entirely different standards for the practice of medicine in the courtroom by making them aware of the behavior and testimony given by "expert" pathologists during a single trial. The defendant at that trial was Jean S. Harris. I submit, however, that we, the medical profession, were also on trial. Would some of the pathologists at that trial have acquitted themselves and the profession more nobly had they known that their behavior and their testimony was to be scrutinized by their peers?

In sum, I have no opinion about the guilt or innocence of Mrs. Harris. I do have an opinion about whether she received an "eminently fair" trial as regards matters of cutaneous histology. To those who say that the cutaneous histology in the trial is irrelevant to whether or not Mrs. Harris shot Dr. Tarnower with intent to murder, I point out that it was the prosecution who made the issue of cutaneous histology relevant when Dr. Roh changed his autopsy report more than nine months after the death of Dr. Tarnower. Who can assess accurately the impact on a jury of eight days of conflicting testimony by pathologists for the prosecution and for the defense? If some, even jurors, claim that the testimony about cutaneous histology played no role in the jury's deliberations, that does not necessarily mean that the implications of the testimony of the pathologists called by the prosecution played no role in the juror's thinking.

The role of cutaneous histology in the trial of Jean Harris and its implications for medicine and the law in the United States should be of concern to the community of physicians. Let it be given careful, reflective, and critical consideration.

Note: The drawings are by Carol Donner, some of them after sketches by Leo Termin, M.D.

The Pathologist in the Courtroom—Peer Review Is Needed*

I have been in a court of law as a pathologist in but a single trial, and that experience had a profoundly disillusioning impact on me. I am told by colleagues who have also appeared in court that my disillusioning experience is not unique. If this is truly the case, there is an urgent need to reassess the role of the physician, and particularly that of the pathologist, in the courtroom. I have drawn on my experiences during the trial of the *People v. Jean S. Harris* for illustrative examples of the types of behavior that I believe should be subjected to peer

*Previously published, under the same title, in the August 1985 edition of *Human Pathology*, Volume 16, No. 8, pp. 761–62. Reprinted with permission from W. B. Saunders Co.

review, just as virtually all other behavior of physicians and their practices in medicine are scrutinized by colleagues.

In brief, Jean Harris, headmistress of the Madeira School in Virginia, shot and killed her unfaithful paramour, Dr. Herman Tarnower, best known as the Scarsdale Diet Doctor. The State contended that Mrs. Harris had shot the doctor in a jealous fit of rage with intent to kill him. The defense claimed that Mrs. Harris had shot Dr. Tarnower by accident when he tried to prevent her from committing suicide. The State claimed that skin from an extended palm of the doctor was found in a bullet wound in his chest, a sign of a "defensive" posture, i.e., the doctor had extended a palm in self-defense, and a bullet fired with intent to kill him had carried his palmar tissue into his chest. Eight pathologists testified about the alleged tissue, two (one of them a dermatopathologist) for the prosecution and six (one of them a dermatopathologist) for the defense. Those testifying for the defense denied that there was any tissue identifiable as palmar in the wound in the chest, claiming that the alleged fragments of palmar tissue were really fragments of connective tissue, probably cartilage.

That the two pathologists who testified for the prosecution should conclude that the fragments of tissue in the wound in the chest were palmar epidermis and the six pathologists for the defense that these fragments were connective tissue is not, in itself, surprising or disturbing. What is alarming to me is the manner in which the evidence for the presence of palmar epidermis in the chest wound was developed by both the prosecutor and the pathologists who testified foro the prosecution.

My indictments of their strategems and procedures are as follows. 1) During the trial, the deputy medical examiner changed his testimony about the number of separate bullets that entered the body of Herman Tarnower from four to three, thereby creating the issue of a "defensive wound" in the palm through which a single bullet passed and then also entered the skin of the chest 2) In the midst of the trial, the deputy medical examiner, after a telephone call from the prosecutor, changed his report of the autopsy findings concerning the wound in the chest: his "new" findings of three small fragments of palmar epidermis in the chest lent support to the prosecution's contention of a palmar wound sustained in self-defense. 3) The deputy medical examiner changed his opinion about the histologic findings in the wound of the chest on five separate occasions. 4) The testimony presented in court by the dermatopathologist for the prosecution about the fragments of tissue in the chest wound differed from statements in his written report. 5) The same dermatopathologist for the prosecution, in a note written to the prosecutor in his own hand, recommended strategy that would "frighten off" other dermatopathologists from testifying in the case. 6) Critical parts of the deputy medical examiner's testimony about cutaneous histology were obviously inaccurate, e.g., he asserted repeatedly that "collagen is a cell" and insisted that collagen has a nucleus, cytoplasm, and cell membrane. 7) The dermatopathologist for the prosecution could not, on his own, present accurately or cogently the histologic criteria for differentiating epithelial from connective tissue ("I would say a very important one is that if we see cells, the cells in the epidermis tend to be more oval-shaped, where cells from collagen, for example, might tend to be very flat and very elongated, sort of spindle-shaped.''). 8) The deputy medical examiner projected photomicrographs to the jury that he and the dermatopathologist for the prosecution acknowledged were out of focus, when the very purpose of the photomicrographs was to convince the jury that three minuscule fragments of tissue were palmar epidermis, not connective tissue. 9) The deputy medical examiner admitted that there were overlays of tissue on the sections that he projected to the jury, but he denied that they represented defects (''It's not a defect. It's the overlay. Defect means absence of something.'')

These and other issues that concern both competence and ethics of pathologists during the trial of Jean Harris have been discussed in greater detail elsewhere.

Unfortunately, all too many physicians, especially pathologists, have become hyposensitized to questionable behavior by doctors in the courtroom. All too often, physicians and society not only fail to condemn, but condone behavior like that just described in the trial of Jean Harris. The typical attitude of many medical colleagues is ''What do you expect?'' My answer is that I expect better. I expect the same kind of behavior that is expected from conscientious pathologists in private laboratories, community hospitals, and universities, i.e., unbiased, professional, strictly truthful behavior. Physicians tend to excuse dubious behavior of other physicians in the courtroom on the grounds that the situation is different there, because, they contend, doctors are not there as practitioners of the healing arts, but as adversaries acting on behalf of litigants and lawyers. I disagree vehemently. Irrespective of the behavior in court of lawyers (who take no oath comparable to that of Hippocrates and who are often fiercely engaged in adversarial relationships), physicians should not be advocates of either a prosecutor or a defense lawyer, but of the unvarnished truth. Physicians should be able to testify with equal neutrality and absolute verity for either side in a dispute, because that testimony should be the truth and only the truth, as they perceive it. It is unthinkable for physicians to play games with the truth. When this is done in universities, physicians are drummed out of the fraternity and forever disgraced. When it is done in the courtroom, physicians are viewed by some colleagues as heroes. This double standard is intolerable, shameful, and unacceptable.

Doctors should treat defendants with the same respect that they show to their patients. For a patient who has several venereal diseases, the obligation of the physician is not to make moral judgments about the behavior of the patient, but to manage the diseases as effectively, expeditiously, and professionally as possible. A defendant deserves no favors from physicians testifying in court but, by the same token, deserves unequivocal commitment to the truth. Defendants should not be pawns in a game played by lawyers, with physician aiding or abetting the players. The defendant deserves professionalism, just that and no more, from physicians in court. Physicians who are called to testify in court are termed ''expert'' witnesses. All too often they are far from expert, and better methods should be devised by the medical profession (not the legal one) to establish criteria for expertness. Defendants, like patients, should be protected.

Medical examiners and prosecutors should function as independent professionals and not as collaborators against litigants. All too often, the game of footsy between the office of the prosecutor and that of the medical examiner is thinly disguised.

In sum, we pathologists have an obligation to ourselves and to our specialty to set standards for behavior in the courtroom that are consistent with our behavior in the rest of our professional lives. That behavior should be elevated and elevating. The behavior of pathologists in the courtroom should be no different from their behavior in the laboratory, but very different from the behavior of all too many lawyers in the courtroom.

Correspondence

The following are responses, in the form of letters to the journal editors, to the foregoing articles. The final letter is Dr. Ackerman's rebuttal to the letter by Dr. Roh.

To the Editor:—Dr. Ackerman's article in the Current Topics section of the August 1984 issue of HUMAN PATHOLOGY concerning the behavior of pathologists as expert witnesses was both pertinent and timely. In the course of my practice in pathology I have appeared as an expert witness on several occasions and will undoubtedly be asked to do so again. In reflecting on these appearances I have discovered an evolution in my own behavior.

My first courtroom appearance was early in my practice. I recall feelings of insecurity and paranoia, as though I were the defendant and my integrity were being questioned. These feelings were undoubtedly communicated to the jury and diluted the effectiveness of what was otherwise knowledgeable testimony. With the passage of time and several additional courtroom appearances, I began to realize my own limitations, as well as the importance of the medical expert's testimony.

I am in complete agreement with Dr. Ackerman that the medical expert should be an unbiased, neutral third party who is called on to explain (teach, if you will) to the jury the significance of some often technical aspect of the case in point. No one who is unprepared, overimpressed with his own importance, feeling threatened, or unable to identify with those being taught (the jury) can be an effective teacher. Accepting the facts that the pathologist is not the one on trial, that the jury is an intelligent group of people expecting from the pathologist a lucid and understandable explanation of some facet of the case that they must consider in its entirety, and that the opposing attorneys basically consider the trial a serious game in which they are competing against each other in a true adversarial relationship redefines the role of the medical expert witness.

Pathology, as a part of medicine, is subjected to uncomfortably close public scrutiny at present. As physicians, we need to demonstrate more than ever that we are caring, concerned, honest, and intelligent people—in short, that we deserve the title of "doctor" in the renaissance context ("learned man"). One of our opportunities for public exposure is the courtroom. Peer review, as Dr. Ackerman suggests, may be a partial answer to appropriate behavior and testimony, but it will not, by itself, suffice. I strongly support his position on the need for physicians to behave in an impartial and intelligent manner when called to testify and thank him for focusing our attention on this aspect of practice that was unforseen by most of us when we chose medicine as a profession.

DAVID J. BLOMBERG, MD
Deaconess Hospital
Evansville, Indiana

To the Editor:—This is to highly commend Dr. Bernard Ackerman for his forceful article (HUM PATHOL 16:761, 1985), concerning the ethics and professionalism—and the lack thereof—of expert witnesses, in particular of pathologists, and their dubious participation in the adversary system practiced by lawyers for both the prosecution and defense. Truer words were never spoken: in fact, this subject, to my knowledge, has never been discussed before. It would be most desirable if that article could be reprinted in more widely read medical journals, such as the *Journal of the American Medical Association*; the *New England Journal of Medicine*; the *Southern Medical Journal*; and, particularly, the *Journal of Forensic Sciences*.

LEO LOWBEER, MD
Clinical Professor of Pathology,
Emeritus
University of Oklahoma School
Of Medicine
Tulsa, Oklahoma

To the Editor:—I have just finished reading the article "The Pathologist in the Courtroom: Peer Review is Needed" by A. Bernard Ackerman (HUM PATHOL 16:761, 1985). While I have insufficient information to comment on the case discussed, I would like to make some general comments in regard to this article. First, I would say that Dr. Ackerman is correct in his belief that pathologists, especially those functioning as medical examiners, should be professional, unbiased, and truthful, as well as true experts when they testify in court. Second, I do not have much sympathy for members of the medical community when they complain about the lack of these attributes in some medical examiner systems.

There are, and have been for a number of years, serious problems with the practicie of forensic pathology in this country. Dr. Ackerman has touched on one of them—the personnel. Until fairly recently, the full-time practice of forensic pathology was a haven for those who were marginally competent in pathology, had personality problems or difficulties in communication, and/or just couldn't get another job. The salaries were typically low, and the working conditions extremely poor. To make things even worse, these pathologists in turn "trained" others, thereby perpetuating the chain of mediocrity and incompetence.

In smaller cities or rural areas, forensic pathology was and is practiced on a part-time basis by hospital pathologists competent in anatomic and clinical pathology, but who often do not know what they are doing in forensic pathology. Unfortunately, they either are unaware of this or like to bask in the publicity that such work can generate. With the recent decline in earnings for pathologists, there is now a financial reason to continue to do forensic work. Some pathologists have built an impressive local reputation by telling the police and prosecutors what they want to hear, reinforcing their "expertise." Dr.

Ackerman may lament the proceedings of the case that he was involved in, but I know of instances in which individuals have been indicted, tried, and, in one recent instance, convicted of murder when the death was a suicide.

While in many areas of this country, the pathologists practicing forensic pathology do not have the education, training, or personality for this specialty, it should be realized that there are many competent pathologists in this field doing excellent work. In fact, the overall quality of physicians now going into forensic pathology has improved dramatically. Unfortunately, in many areas of the country, individuals, whether good or incompetent, are working under poor medicolegal laws, in inadequate facilities, without proper equipment, and with insufficient personnel and funding. This is due, in part, to a lack of support for good medicolegal systems by the medical community, coupled with indifference on the part of politicians and the judiciary. This medical community, as a general rule, does not care about the competency of a medicolegal system as long as it is not directly affected. Most pathology training programs still do not provide sufficient exposure to forensic pathology to their residents. Pathologists in private practice cannot understand why a pathologist would work so hard at such a distasteful occupation, in poor working conditions, for so little money. Many academic pathologists share the same feelings, and, in addition, cannot understand a system the opposite of their own, where the autopsies are performed by the most rather than the least senior pathologists. Academic institutions generally have very little idea as to how a medical examiner system functions, or of staffing and the equipment that is necessary.

Research in forensic medicine is minimal, as there is virtually no money available for it. When money for research is obtainable, it is often for obscure entities and for reasons of medical, not medicolegal interest (the two are not necessarily identical).

I would like to end this letter on an optimistic note. There are many good medical examiner's offices and many good forensic pathologists. The quality of the pathologists going into forensic pathology is increasing, as is the support by the political community in many areas.

VINCENT J. M. DIMAIO, MD
Chief Medical Examiner
San Antonio, Texas

To the Editor:—Doctor A. Bernard Ackerman's experience (HUM PATHOL 16:761, 1985) raises an issue that forensic pathologists in particular should address but that has gone largely ignored. Implicit in his discussion is the reality that "the game of footsy between the office of prosecutor and that of the medical examiner" is rife with opportunities for prostitution of opinion. Whether or not such prostitution occurs depends entirely on the ethics of the prosecutor and/or the pathologist witness, and I feel very fortunate not to have seen it personally until this year, after having spent 15 years performing medicolegal autopsies for a combined total of ten different prosecutorial jurisdictions. When one sees deliberate distortion or concealment of the truth and a possibly innocent man (or woman) serve one or two life sentences, one has a profound sense of disgust. When the misinformation is provided by a physician and encouraged by an attorney charged by the community with the responsibility of administering "justice," the disgust is greater for the reasons Dr. Ackerman has discussed. HUMAN

PATHOLOGY should be congratulated for including a paper on an ethical issue in the pathology literature.

PETER J. STEPHENS, MD
Davenport, Iowa

To the Editor:—I would like to commend Dr. A. Bernard Ackerman for his excellent article, "The Pathologist in the Courtroom: Peer Review is Needed" (HUM PATHOL 16:761, 1985). Since Dr. Ackerman's article relates only to a single case, one may argue it away as a rare occurrence. Unfortunately, it is not as rare as one might think. Although, in most cases, the medical expert will render an honest opinion, in too many cases this is not so. It has been my experience in testifying numerous times in medical examiner cases and in private civil and criminal cases that such practices are, indeed, quite common and very frustrating. In many instances the information presented by the expert to the jury is either pure nonsense, incorrect medical facts, nonfactual scientific jargon, facts taken out of context to confuse, or outright ludicrous. It is very difficult to understand why some experts with excellent credentials will testify as they do. In this regard, one must wonder whether it is done solely for monetary purposes. If this is correct, then they are no different from "scientific hookers" or "hired guns" who use their impressive credentials and double talk to support the allegations of the lawyers they represent . . . "you pay, I say." One must understand that I am not talking about differences in opinion between experts, since such differences may merely reflect an interpretation derived from a different perspective, from personal experience, or from greater or lesser cognitive ability or mental acuity.

This practice constitutes a serious problem. The question is simple—what can be done to stop these practices? The answer, however, is not so simple, but one thing is certain. Some type of peer review must be implemented to prevent miscarriages of justice.

FREDERICK T. ZUGIBE, MD, PhD
Chief Medical Examiner
County of Rockland, New York

To the Editor:—The single case presented by Ackerman served as an appropriate illustration of your editorial slug line in the same issue. The publication by your journal of [what is at best] an ad hominem attack on a (deputy) medical examiner is quite surprising. No supporting material is presented by Ackerman to support his allegations. No rebuttal [by the one maligned] was provided in the journal. The issue of whether the questioned wound was an entry or reentry wound cannot be evaluated independently with the material presented to Ackerman. [At worst, HUMAN PATHOLOGY has aided in the publication of a libel.] Ackerman cannot ignore that his paid testimony for the defense was subjected to peer review in its appropriate sense and a jury found against the defendant in *People v. Harris*. The state's problem with the defense expert [who lies] has been addressed well elsewhere.

This office, for example, is funded by the State of Georgia. Liberal rules of discovery assure access to findings of the medical examiners as well as the scientists of the crime laboratory. Consultants are utilized where appropriate. Physical evidence is retained and is available for discussion and review by outside experts. Pretrial conferences are held with both prosecutors and defense counsel when requested by both parties. At those conferences hypothetical scenarios are explored. Where physical evidence does not support the state, prosecution should not follow. Adequate trial preparation benefits both the state and the defendant. Medical examiners in this office do not accept fees when testifying for criminal defendants. The generalization by Ackerman regarding the intimacy of medical examiners and prosecutors is unfortunate.

Forensic pathology is a distinct subspecialty of pathology, with appropriate requirements for certification by the American Board of Pathology. There are too few of us to meet the actual needs of the public to investigate independently the causes of all deaths. The use of other physicians is a necessity, and how few are the universities that provide any training in forensic pathology. Criteria for "expertness," as in other areas of medicine, must include training and experience. Should every anatomic pathologist participate successfully in the PIP program of the College of American pathologists? Does Ackerman have other criteria in mind?

Peer review is applied most appropriately in a courtroom. There, 12 persons sift fact and apply judgment conditioned by experience and community standards to arrive at the truth of a situation. Expert review as proffered by Ackerman falls short of that achievement (dermatopathologists divided 1–1 in *People v. Harris*).

The critical question is who is telling the truth. Integrity cannot be legislated.

KENNETH ALONSO, MD, FACP
Chief Medical Examiner
Divison of Forensic Sciences
Georgia Bureau of Investigation
Decatur, Georgia

Dr. Ackerman responds:—The only libel is Dr. Kenneth Alonso's assertion about my "paid testimony." I neither asked for nor received any payment whatsoever for my testimony—*A. Bernard Ackerman, MD*

Note: The letter to which Dr. Ackerman responded contained the words that appear in brackets. Dr. Alonso subsequently requested the deletion of these words, and they appear here to clarify the response.

To the Editor:—I would like to reply to and make a few comments on the article "The Pathologist in The Courtroom: Peer Review Is Needed" (HUM PATHOL 16:761, 1985). As the Deputy Medical Examiner-Forensic Pathologist involved in *People v. Jean Harris*, I find it disturbing to read an article by a physician inexperienced in forensic pathology on the practice of legal medicine and the judicial system.

Dr. Herman Tarnower, a respected cardiologist and the author of *Scarsdale Diet Book*, was awakened in the middle of the night and shot at five times by Mrs. Jean S. Harris. Three bullets were recovered in the body and two at the scene. The defense claimed that it was a "tragic accident." There was a protracted trial, and Mrs. Harris was found guilty of murder. After the trial one of the jurors stated, "We reenacted the situation. There were 20 ways it (accidental shooting) could have happened but not the way the defense described it."

During the initial investigation I visited the scene as a deputy medical examiner with forensic scientists and a ballistic specialist to evaluate and reconstruct the events. It was our opinion that Dr. Tarnower had been awakened by Mrs. Harris and had subsequently sat on the ledge of the bed while she stood in front of him. He had then seen a gun in her left hand pointing at him. He had raised his right hand to ward off the gun but received a close contact bullet wound in the palmar surface of his hand; the bullet had then reentered his right anterior upper chest, forming a linear trajectory from her gun to his outstretched hand and chest. The four shots fired thereafter had caused his death as a result of multiple internal injuries.

I initially testified at the trial about the cause of death and the above-mentioned "defensive gesture." During the trial, at the suggestion of a defense expert, I reexamined the microscopic slide of Dr. Tarnower's chest wound prepared at the time of autopsy and found three tiny fragments of palmar epidermis, gun powder, and fibers from his pajamas carried by the penetrating bullet and left in the bullet track in the subcutaneous adipose tissue, which provided additional support for my opinion. I consulted colleagues, including a dermatopathologist who is a professor of dermatopathology and the author of many books and articles. All agreed that the section showed palmar epidermis.

I then issued a supplemental report as to the additional discovery. The defense then hired six pathologists, including a dermatopathologist. All said that the material was not palmar epidermis but could not agree as to what it was.

The following are my answers to the author's "indictments":

1. The author claims that I changed my testimony as to the number of bullets that entered Dr. Tarnower's body from four to three. Obviously, the author does not understand the forensic autopsy description and interpretation, including the number of bullets, number of bullet wounds, and number of bullet tracks. If the victim had four wounds and three bullets were found in the body, one bullet obviously had to cause an extra wound by reentering the body, especially since the trajectory was a linear path, the primary target was in close contact, and the secondary target showed an irregular perforating entrance wound with minimum penetration.

2. The author claims that I changed the autopsy findings concerning the wound in the chest that contained palmar tissue. Medicine is an informative science; if new evidence and test results are found, it is common practice to issue a supplemental report. The additional report was not a change of findings, but rather a truer presentation of the facts as I believed them to be at the time.

3. The author claims that I changed my opinion about the histologic findings in the wound of the chest. I discovered palmar tissue in the chest wound in the microscopic slide, after which I consulted my colleagues and a professor of dermatopathology and issued a supplemental report. Not to do so would have been an omission of my duty as a medical examiner.

4. The author claims that my lack of knowledge of collagen was a critical error. The critical issue was the existence of palmar epidermis in the wound, not collagen. During the trial I was questioned by the defense lawyer and the author extensively on such subjects as intercellular bridges and their ultrastructural morphology, definitions of necrosis and change, collagen fiber and its morphology, and embryology, the nature of the fibroblast and its function, the definition of the tonofibril and its electron microscopic features, and the polarization of tissue samples. The fact is that palmar epidermis was found in the victim's anterior chest.

5. The author claims that photomicrographs shown to the jury were out of focus. The perimeter of a few photomicrographs at higher magnification were slightly out of focus; however, the points of interest were clearly and accurately depicted. All of the photo-

micrographs admitted as evidence in court were used by the prosecution as well as the defense. All of the details were seen and explained to the jury by both sides.

6. The author claims that there were overlays of tissue on the sections. Defense and the author insisted that this was a defect. These were a few artifacts or "floaters," not a defect.

7. The three remaining comments applied to the testifying dermatopathologist, and therefore I cannot respond to them.

These are answers to the author's indictments. The autopsy report, microscopic slides, and photomicrographs are still available for examination as public records kept in the medical examiner's office.

The author also testified and was cross-examined, while I was excluded from the courtroom. The following are a few excerpts from his testimony:

Answer: One doesn't have nuclei there (palmar epidermis). They (nuclei) are the findings of cartilage. They (nuclei) are not found in the skin.

Question: There is a big difference between the cornified layer of the anterior chest and the palm. Isn't there?

Answer: Theoretically that is correct, but the fact is we don't know.

Answer: The cornified layer polarizes more intensely than the fibrocartilage.

The author insists that physicians should be able to testify with equal neutrality and absolute verity for either side in a dispute, and yet the author writes articles illustrated by erroneous schematic drawings when actual photographs are available. Furthermore, reprints of the same article were given to Mrs. Harris in jail so that she could mail the copy to Dr. Tarnower's surviving family.

The author insists that the testimony should be the truth and only the truth.

The Court: The notes [about the case] are in your office, are they, Doctor?

Witness: Either in my home or in my office, one or the other.

After the prosecutor asked for a recess to get the notes.

Witness: I may well have tossed those notes out.

It is unfortunate that a well-respected dermatopathologist who testified for "the first time ever" and had "practically never" examined tissue sections that involved a bullet wound criticizes a forensic pathologist, dermatopathologist, prosecutor, criminal investigator, and the judicial system. The role of the physician in court is to tell the truth and express an opinion with a reasonable degree of medical certainty. The verdict should be made by the jury and the court. All too often inexperienced physicians take a verdict contrary to their testimony as a personal defeat. Yes, I do believe that peer review is needed, and let each speciality of medicine and law remain in its own domain.

LOUIS ROH, MD
Forensic Pathologist Deputy Medical
Examiner
Westchester County Medical
Examiner's Office
Valhalla, New York

To the Editor:—This letter is in response to the Letter to the Editor (HUMAN PATHOLOGY 17:326–327, 1986 March) by Louis Roh, M.D., Deputy Medical Examiner of Westchester County. Although I could rebut each of Dr. Roh's inaccuracies, I will confine this reply to his ''quotations'' from the transcripts, every one of which he has misrepresented.

1) In his Letter, Dr. Roh wrote:

The following are a few excerpts from his [Ackerman's] testimony:
Answer: One doesn't have nuclei there [palmar epidermis]. They [nuclei] are not found in the skin.

What the transcript actually states on page 6459 about the colloquy between Assistant District Attorney Georoge Bolen and me is:

Question: Did you also read the subsequent report, or I guess it's called the addendum to the histological examination which Dr. Roh prepared and signed on January 8th of this year?

Answer: I did.

Question: Would you comment, please, as to whether or not that report is consistent with your own findings and opinion?

Answer: It is in part consistent with my findings, but in part it is not and is not consistent with my conclusion. Dr. Roh insists that there are irregular empty spaces containing nuclei [sic] material. That is consistent with my finding. But those findings are not the findings in the *cornified layer* (italics mine) of the palmar skin or any skin that is normal. One doesn't have nuclei there and no spaces around it. They are the findings of cartilage. They are not found [in the cornified layer] in the skin.

2) Another excerpt from the transcript inaccurately attributed to me by Dr. Roh is:

Question: There is a big difference between the cornified layer of the anterior chest and the palm. Isn't there?

Answer: Theoretically that is correct, but the fact is we don't know.

In truth, the transcript on pages 6502 and 6503 reads:

Question: There is a big difference between the cornified layer of the anterior chest and the palm. Isn't there?

Answer: That's correct.

Question: I mean that palm is so much thicker than the anterior chest because of the nature of the beast, what the hand is called upon to do?

Answer: Teleologically (italics mine), that is correct. But the fact is we don't know. It's thicker.

3) Without first posing the necessary question, Dr. Roh attributed this answer to me as if it were a quotation directly from the transcript:

Answer: The cornified layer polarizes more intensely than the fibrocartilage.

In fact, the transcript on pages 6518 and 6519 records the dialogue precisely as follows:

Question: If I understand correctly, Doctor, with regard to the polarization and the joint examination that you and your colleagues, Dr. Roh and Dr. Paparo and so forth, did, you polarized the fragments and compared them on the one hand with actual tissue preserved at autopsy from Dr. Tarnower's cornified layer of the palm, and on the other, with what Dr. Roh furnished you as fibrocartilage. Is that correct?

Answer: That's correct.

Question: At that point, without telling us about anybody else, will you tell us your observations and conclusions in that regard?

Answer: My observations were that the cornified layer polarized more intensely than the fibrocartilage and the three fragments and the fibrocartilage had approximately the same intensity of polarization.

4) Dr. Roh took the following "quotations" completely out of context and thus gave an entirely erroneous sense of the matter in point:

The Court: The notes [about the case] are in your office, are they, Doctor?

Witness: Either in my home or in my office, one or the other.

After the prosecution asked for a recess to get the notes.

Witness: I may well have tossed those notes out.

In fact, the notes of my findings about the three fragments in the skin in the wound of the chest of Dr. Tarnower were jotted down (as is my custom in preparation for later transcription of them by my secretary) on the back of a manila envelope immediately after I had examined the histologic sections in the medical examiner's office. Those original notes were then indeed typed. The typed notes were discarded, but the original ones were preserved and were in the hands of Judge Leggett from the time that he requested them of me until the end of the trial. What the transcript actually records on pages 6467, 6468, 6473, 6474, and 6492 is as follows:

The Court: The only reason the district attorney would want to look at this is just to make sure, if these notes are available, that your testimony is essentially similar to this.

If you had overlooked a material fact inadvertently and it was recorded in your notes, that might or might not have significance to the attorneys. I will tell you what I could like you to do. First of all, make a good faith effort to call your office now to see if in fact those notes are there. I am sure they are probably thumbnail notes—

The Witness: They were written on the back of a manila envelope.

The Court: They are the kind of notes I would make under certain circumstances to just remind you for 20 minutes.

The Witness: If they are there, they will be there. My secretary will know.

[My secretary did have the notes and read them by telephone to Judge Leggett, who transmitted them to the court reporter who, in turn, recorded them on pages 6470–6472 of the transcript.]

Question: Did you at any time on Thursday dictate any type of report, formal written report?

Answer: I had my secretary type for me notes, the very notes that are on my manila envelope.

Question: Did your secretary do that Thursday?

Answer: Yesterday.

Question: Where are those typewritten notes now?

Answer: I took them home with me to study those and then I tossed them out. They are the same notes that are on the back on the manila envelope.

The Court: I have satisfied myself that you are not a professional witness who should have known to bring these notes along, and while Mr. Aurnou [the lawyer for Mrs. Harris] should have told you, he didn't. I made up my mind in my own judgment that this was not deliberate, and certainly you should not be penalized by having to run around more. On the other hand, to guarantee or to assure as far as possible the integrity of what we have done here, I am going to direct that you forward up here your original notes just as they exist without any alteration or touching of them at all.

Witness Ackerman: Fine.

The Court: That would require you mailing me the original envelope, and I want it done forthwith, as soon as you can.

Witness Ackerman: As soon as I get back to my office.

Dr. Roh concluded his letter by advising readers that "The role of the physician in court is to tell the truth and express an opinion with a reasonable degree of medical certainty. The verdict should be made by the jury and the court." Of course a jury must be the ultimate arbiter, but in order for a jury to judge fairly it must be given accurate information. Its judgment must be based upon a firm foundation of facts. When pathologists give flawed evidence to juries, they sabotage the jury system by making it impossible for juries of lay men and women to assess medical testimony intelligently and thus to render just verdicts.

A. BERNARD ACKERMAN

5. The Validity of Urine Alcohol Analysis in Drunk Drivers

Charles L. Winek, Ph.D. and Francis M. Esposito, Ph.D.

INTRODUCTION

Ethanol is the chemical agent most commonly found in persons charged with "driving under the influence." Statutes exist in each state prohibiting the operation of a motor vehicle while under the influence of alcohol. Penalties vary, but all include revocation or suspension of a drivers' license, fines and/or incarceration.

State Statutes

Scientific investigations have shown a relationship between a subject's blood alcohol concentration (BAC) and impairment of abilities necessary to operate a motor vehicle safely[1]. In turn, each state has adopted legislation governing the operation of a motor vehicle while under the influence of an intoxicating liquor. Most states define a person with 0.05 percent or less of alcohol by weight in his or her blood or breadth as not being under the influence of an intoxicating liquor. A person whose test reveals an alcohol level in excess of 0.05 percent, but less than 0.10 percent, may or may not be under the influence, and the test results should be considered along with other evidence, such as sobriety tests. Finally, if a test shows a BAC of 0.10 percent or more, it is presumed that the person is under the influence of alcohol.

The above provisions were first issued in the Uniform Vehicle Code of 1945. Since then, every state has adopted statutes with similar provisions. Twenty-seven states still use presumptive or *primae facie* clauses, through which defendants testing above 0.10 percent can be acquitted of charges of raising doubt as to their having been under the influence. A newer statute, known as the *Per Se* law, has been enacted in 20 states. This statute specifically prohibits driving with a BAC of 0.10 percent or more. Oregon has followed the example of many European countries by setting the level for intoxication at 0.08 percent. Several states use two levels for prosecution, a lower level for presumption and a higher level as *Per Se*. Blood levels around 0.05 percent are being considered by some states as upper statutory limits for underage drinkers.

Chemical Tests

Chemical tests for intoxication estimate the amount of alcohol absorbed into the brain by analyzing blood, breath, urine, or other bodily substances. Blood and breath are the specimens routinely submitted for ethanol quantitation and interpretation of alcohol intoxication. Every state authorizes the use of blood or breath as test specimens. In lieu of these specimens, 16 states permit submitting urine and 17 states permit submitting urine or some other bodily fluid (such as saliva). Although some state statutes provide for alcohol analysis of urine, a portion of these states will not analyze urine because legislation has failed to establish rules and regulations regarding the procedure of abstraction or means of measurement of alcohol content in urine. Yet, other states will analyze urine, since legislation permits it to be submitted even though procedures for collection are not detailed.

Toxicologists disagree as to the existence of a definite relationship between blood and urine alcohol concentrations. That is, will a chemical test of urine accurately reflect the corresponding blood level when urine is collected? Should more than one sample be submitted and, if so, what is the time limit for the second specimen? Finally, what urine level should be used for charging people with driving under the influence? This article will address each of these questions.

ALCOHOL DISTRIBUTION

Alcohol is absorbed into the blood through the stomach and the walls of the small intestines. Once absorbed, alcohol is distributed by the blood to body tissues and fluids in proportion to their water content and blood supply. When absorption and distribution are complete, equilibrium is achieved and the alcohol concentration in the body tissues and fluids is directly proportional to their water content.

Urine is a waste fluid excreted by the kidneys as blood is filtered by the kidneys. The concentration of alcohol in urine as it is being formed and as it passes through the ureter on its way to the bladder corresponds to the blood concentration. The urine concentration will be about 1.3 times higher than the blood when it is being manufactured because the water content of urine is more

Figure 5.1

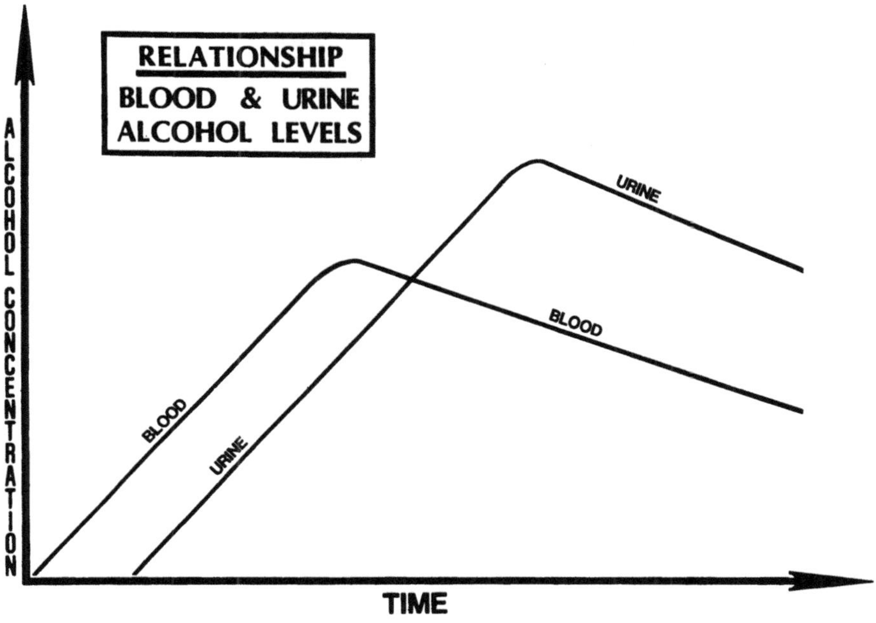

than blood and alcohol dissolves in a fluid in proportion to its water content. But before alcohol appears in the urine it must first be absorbed into the blood and excreted into the urine—thus, urine levels lag behind blood levels. Blood levels rise when the rate of absorption of alcohol from the gastrointestinal tract is greater than the rate of dissipation (from metabolism and excretion). The concentration of ethanol in the urine in the ureter parallels the rise and fall of blood levels (Figure 5.1). Hence a sample of urine as it is manufactured will accurately reflect a blood alcohol level at that moment (in the same manner that a breath specimen reflects a blood level).

After urine accumulates in the bladder over a period of time, it is then a composite of urine of higher and lower levels of alcohol content. In addition, any urine in the bladder at the time of urine formation and subsequent passage to the bladder will dilute the filtered urine and lower the urine alcohol concentration. On the other hand, failure to urinate for extended periods will result in accumulation of excreted alcohol in the bladder. Thus, the concentration of alcohol in urine in the bladder may not reflect a blood level at the time the urine is collected, especially if one has not voided for a considerable time.

Urine/Blood Ratios

The ratio of the amount of alcohol in the urine compared to that in the blood after the alcohol is distributed and equilibrium exists is known as the distribution ratio. The urine/blood ratio, based on the water content of the specimens, is 1.2 or 1.3 to 1. But several studies using autopsy specimens have shown varying average ratios. Our laboratory found a urine/blood ratio of 1.57 [2], while others have reported ratios of 1.16 [3] and 1.28 [4].

To calculate a blood alcohol level from a given urine alcohol level, the distribution ratio is used as in the following equation:

$$\frac{\text{urine alcohol concentration}}{\text{distribution ratio of urine/blood}} = \text{blood alcohol concentration}$$

Suppose the urine level is 133 mg percent. The calculated blood level would range from 85 mg percent to 115 mg percent, depending on the average distribution ratio chosen (133 mg% ÷ 1.57 = 85 mg% and 133 mg% ÷ 1.16 = 115 mg%). This puts the predicted blood level either above or below the legal limit of 100 mg percent.

Each of the following postmortem studies also revealed a very wide range of individual urine/blood alcohol ratios. We found the individual ratios to be from 0.07 to 21.0. Thus, from a given urine alcohol level, the corresponding blood level would encompass an enormous range of levels if the individual ratios are used. For example, again using a urine level of 133 mg percent, the calculated blood levels could range from 6 mg percent to an impossible level of 1,900 mg percent (133 mg% ÷ 21.0 = 6 mg% and 133 mg% ÷ 0.07 = 1,900 mg%).

Why such a large range of individual urine/blood ratios? The principal reason is that these studies used postmortem samples, and a number of uncontrollable circumstances can influence these ratios. But similar factors can occur in the case of the living individual that may also result in wide urine/blood ratios, should a single urine specimen be collected from the bladder. For example, the stage of alcohol absorption, whether at the time of death or when a urine sample is taken from a living person, will influence the ratio. As explained earlier, during alcohol absorption from the gastrointestinal tract, the urine level lags behind the blood level since alcohol must first be absorbed and excreted from the blood before it appears in the urine. If a urine sample is collected during the absorption phase, the urine/blood ration will be low. If the bladder is already full, at the time urine containing the alcohol is excreted into the bladder, the alcohol will be diluted further, lowering the urine/blood ratio. This may be the reason for some of the low urine/blood alcohol ratios listed in Table 5.1. Conversely, if a long period of time exists between one's last drink and when he or she voids, then a high urine/blood ratio may be expected, as shown in Table 5.2. Such instances would occur if the person has died while asleep or gone into a coma. Alcohol in the blood will continue to be excreted into the urine until death, thus accumulating large amounts of alcohol in the unemptied bladder.

Table 5.1
Postmortem Examples Where Urine Alcohol Content/Blood Alcohol Content is Less Than 1.3

BLOOD ALCOHOL	URINE ALCOHOL	URINE/ BLOOD	% DIFFERENCE
0.05	0.04	0.90	-20
0.06	0.02	0.33	-66
0.05	0.01	0.20	-80
0.04	0.02	0.50	-50
0.05	0.01	0.20	-80
0.07	0.02	0.29	-71
0.06	0.02	0.33	-67
0.09	0.01	0.11	-79
0.07	0.01	0.14	-86
0.05	0.01	0.20	-80
0.22	0.03	0.14	-86
0.57	0.15	0.26	-74
0.10	0.01	0.10	-90
0.45	0.18	0.40	-60
0.14	0.06	0.43	-57
0.16	0.03	0.19	-81
0.15	0.01	0.07	-93
0.14	0.01	0.07	-93
0.10	0.02	0.20	-80
0.18	0.03	0.17	-83

CORRELATION OF URINE ALCOHOL TO BLOOD ALCOHOL

As demonstrated by autopsy studies, precaution should be observed when trying to correlate a urine alcohol level to a blood alcohol level if only one urine sample is submitted. Investigators disagree as to the reliability of predicting blood levels from a random specimen of urine from living individuals. Morgan [5] simultaneously analyzed blood and the first urine sample submitted, and concluded that it is unsatisfactory to calculate blood levels from one urine sample. He found that the urine and calculated blood levels correspond in 44.7 percent of the cases, while 43.7 percent showed calculated values less than actual and 11.6 percent had values higher than calculated. Heise [6] states "the concentration of alcohol in urine in the post-absorptive phase is suitable for the making of a judgement regarding impairment of the individual providing the specimen." Both investigations analyzed the first urine specimen submitted. Although Biasotti and Valentine [7] did not do a direct urine to blood correlation study, they believe a second urine sample is a reliable alternative to blood alcohol determinations.

Haggard and his associates [8] also investigated the use of urine as a specimen for chemical testing for intoxication. Their findings were as follows: During the absorption of alcohol from the gastrointestinal tract, the urine level lagged behind

Table 5.2
Postmortem Examples Where Urine Alcohol Content/Blood Alcohol Content is Greater Than 1.3

BLOOD ALCOHOL	URINE ALCOHOL	URINE/ BLOOD	% DIFFERENCE
0.01	0.05	5.00	+80
0.07	0.15	2.14	+93
0.03	0.10	3.33	+70
0.06	0.50	8.33	+88
0.03	0.25	8.33	+88
0.01	0.04	4.00	+75
0.04	0.10	2.50	+60
0.01	0.12	12.00	+92
0.01	0.21	21.00	+95
0.10	0.21	2.10	+52
0.10	0.26	2.60	+62
0.14	0.29	2.07	+51
0.10	0.34	3.40	+71
0.13	0.30	2.31	+57
0.18	0.34	1.89	+47
0.03	0.15	5.00	+93
0.01	0.19	19.00	+95
0.05	0.27	5.40	+81
0.22	0.40	1.81	+45
0.16	0.24	2.40	+58

the blood level for the first hour after ingestion (Table 5.3). An hour after ingestion, the blood alcohol maximum was reached after which the blood level falls due to metabolism and excretion of alcohol. The urine level also maximizes and falls. A close correlation was achieved between blood alcohol levels and urine levels after the first hour by having the subjects empty their bladders, discarding the specimen and examining another specimen voided 30 minutes later (Table 5.3). However, if the urine is allowed to accumulate in the bladder, then the correlation is not as good. For example, when urine was allowed to collect in the bladder for 4 hours or more rather than the half-hour intervals, the predicted blood values from urine levels were 0.169 percent, and 0.150 percent, when in actuality the blood concentrations were 0.129 percent, 0.078 percent, and 0.037 percent, respectively. However, in each of these cases, once the bladder was emptied and a urine sample submitted one half hour later, the predicted blood values were 0.116 percent, 0.069 percent, and 0.34 percent, each of which is very close to the actual corresponding blood values of 0.115 percent, 0.055 percent, and 0.030 percent, respectively. Hence, when urine accumulates in the bladder awhile, a blood prediction is invalid; but, once the bladder is emptied of its contents, a sample collected one half hour later will more accurately reflect a blood level.

Ordinarily, urine does not accumulate in the bladder, since alcohol has a diuretic effect and the intake of large quantities of fluid induces frequent uri-

Table 5.3
Concentration of Alcohol in Blood and Urine

TIME AFTER INGESTION OF ALCOHOL-HOURS	CONCENTRATION OF ALCOHOL IN BLOOD %	PREDICTED BLOOD LEVELS FROM URINE VOIDED AT INTERVALS OF:				
		½ Hour	2 Hours	4 Hours	6 Hours	7 Hours
½	0.152	0.037				
1	0.193	0.163				
1½	0.191	0.192				
2	0.185	0.188	0.171			
2½	0.171	0.177				
3	0.160	0.165				
3½	0.141	0.146				
4	0.129	0.133	0.171	0.169		
4½	0.115	0.111		0.116		
5	0.103	0.109				
5½	0.091	0.100				
6	0.078	0.082	0.106		0.158	
6½	0.066	0.070			0.069	
7	0.057	0.062				
7½	0.049	0.051				
8	0.037	0.043	0.057			0.150
8½	0.030	0.033				0.034
9	0.023	0.026				
9½	0.016	0.021				
10	0.007	0.012	0.024			
10½	0.003	0.005				
11	0.000	0.003				

Table taken and modified from: *Journal of the American Medical Association*, Volume 115, Number 20, (1940).

nation. But diureses may not occur in everyone, and large amounts of fluid are not taken when "shots" of hard liquor are imbibed, so retention of urine is possible.

Problems of Urinalysis for Alcohol

In the study done by Haggard *et. al.* [8], it was shown that urine can be a reliable estimate of the alcohol concentration in blood only in the post-absorptive phase and only if the subject completely empties his bladder, so that this specimen may be discarded and another specimen voided and examined about 30 minutes later. However, urinalysis is fraught with problems. The subject may intentionally not completely empty his bladder the first time, thereby making any subsequent samples possibly invalid. Also, one often cannot urinate in the specified time after the first specimen has been discarded. To insure validity of the specimen, someone must supervise the collection of the sample so that it is not tampered with by adding water and that, indeed, it is a urine sample and not a water sample.

Sixteen states permit a urine specimen to be submitted for alcohol analysis in lieu of blood or breath, but many of these states do not have regulations regarding the procedure for urine collection. As shown through autopsy and antemortem studies, only a urine specimen collected about 30 minutes after complete voiding will reflect a blood alcohol level. If regulations do not exist regarding proper guidelines for urine collection, then the urine alcohol content may not accurately reflect the blood level at the time urine is collected for analysis.

An additional problem with state laws is that few actually list the correct statutory limit for alcohol content in urine. Based on distribution studies and on the water content of urine and blood, the urine/blood ratio is about 1.3. Thus, a urine level of 0.13 percent is equivalent to a blood level of 0.10 percent. It is incorrect to list 0.10 percent as the statutory limit for urine since this value is equivalent to a blood level of 0.077 percent, as follows:

$$\frac{\text{urine}}{\text{blood}} = 1.3, \text{ or } \frac{\text{urine}}{1.3} = \text{blood, and } \frac{0.10\%}{1.3} = 0.077\%$$

Some states use distribution ratios of 1.33 and 1.49, so urine statutory limits would be 0.133 percent and 0.149 percent, respectively. Because states express blood statutory limits as 0.10 grams/100 ml, and oftentimes a breath limit of 0.10 grams/210 liters of breath, urine limits can be expressed as 0.10 grams/67 ml of urine or 0.10 grams/75.3 ml of urine when using urine/blood distribution ratios of 1.33 and 1.49, respectively.

Recommendations for Urinalysis of Alcohol

Urine in the bladder is a composite sample of alcohol excreted over time. To avoid the problems of dilution or accumulation of alcohol in the bladder, the subject must empty his bladder and the specimen should be discarded. A sample obtained 20 to 30 minutes later will more accurately reflect a blood level, since urine being manufactured correlates with blood in alcohol content until the urine is mixed with urine accumulated in the bladder over a period of time. But one should be sure the subject is in the post-absorptive phase; otherwise, the predicted blood value will be lower than the actual value. Therefore, an additional urine specimen should be submitted about 30 minutes after the first submitted sample. If the second urine sample is lower in alcohol than the first, the individual is in the post-absorptive phase, and the urine value will reflect the blood value. However, if the second urine sample has a higher alcohol value, then the person is in the absorption phase, and any blood predictions from the first sample will be lower than actual (in the defendant's favor).

Once the urine value is obtained, it is divided by the distribution ratio of urine to blood. The dividend is the blood alcohol concentration at the time the urine sample was submitted. Which distribution ratio value to use is a matter of debate. As previously mentioned, autopsy cases show this value to range from 1.16 to 1.57. The value most used is the average ratio of 1.35. When urine concentrations are 200 mg percent or higher, the distribution chosen for conversions is not as important as when the urine level is near 130 mg percent. As demonstrated earlier, a urine level of 133 mg percent could correspond to a blood level of 85 mg percent to 115 mg percent depending on the distribution ratio used in the calculations. The subject in one case is legally intoxicated and not in the other. A urine value of 200 mg percent will put the subject above the statutory limit of 0.10 percent no matter which distribution ratio is used. For example, calculated blood concentrations of 172 mg percent and 127 mg percent would correspond to a urine level of 200 mg percent using the distribution ratios of 1.16 and 1.57, respectively (200 mg percent ÷ 1.16 = 172 mg percent and 200 mg percent ÷ 1.57 = 127 mg percent). With the frequently used ratio of 1.3, the predicted blood level is 154 mg percent (200 mg percent ÷ 1.3 = 154 mg percent). Hence, a urine concentration above 200 mg percent will correspond to a blood level greater than 100 mg percent.

To avoid calculations to presumed blood levels, statutory limits of urine alcohol should exist, as they do for blood, such as 0.13 percent (0.13 grams of alcohol per 100 ml of urine). A second urine sample taken after the first voiding of the bladder should be used for analysis.

Finally, to insure validity of the urine specimen, a police officer must supervise the collection of the sample to assure the specimen's authenticity.

SUMMARY

Blood and breath are the specimens of choice for determining alcohol levels. A random urine specimen may not reflect a blood level because of the influences due to the stage of absorption, the quantity of urine in the bladder, and the frequency of urination. A urine sample may accurately reflect a blood level only

30 minutes after the bladder is completely emptied. Individual states that permit urinalysis for alcohol must provide procedures for sample collection and statutory limit levels.

REFERENCES

1. *American Medical Association*, ''Alcohol and the Impaired Driver,'' (1970), Chicago, IL, 27–34.

2. Winek, C. L., Murphy, K. L. and Winek, T. A., ''The Unreliability of Using a Urine Ethanol Concentration to Predict a Blood Ethanol Concentration,'' *Forensic Science International*, vol. 25, 1984, 277–81.

3. Backer, R. D., Pisano, R. V. and Sopher, I. M., ''The Comparison of Alcohol Concentrations in Postmortem Fluids and Tissues,'' *Journal of Forensic Science* 1980, 327–31.

4. Kaye, S. and Cardona, E., ''Errors of Converting a Urine Alcohol Value Into a Blood Alcohol Value,'' *American Journal of Clinical Pathology*, vol. 52, 5, 1969, 577–84.

5. Morgan, W. H. D., ''Concentrations of Alcohol in Samples of Blood and Urine Taken at the Same Time,'' *Journal of Forensic Science*, vol. 5, 1965, 15–21.

6. Heise, H. A., ''Concentrations of Alcohol in Samples of Blood and Urine Taken at the Same Time,'' *Journal of Forensic Science*, vol. 12, 4 1967, 454–62.

7. Biasotti, A. A. and Valentine, T. E., ''Blood Alcohol Concentration Determined from Urine Samples as a Practical Equivalent or Alternative to Blood and Breath Alcohol Tests,'' *Journal of Forensic Science*, vol. 30, 1, 1985, 194–207.

8. Haggard, H. W., Greenberg, L. A., Corroll, R. P., and Miller, D. P., ''The Use of Urine in the Chemical Test for Intoxication,'' *Journal of the American Medical Association*, vol. 115, 20, 1940, 1680–83.

6. Low-back Pain—Diagnosis, Treatment, and Medicolegal Considerations

Richard Arnold Silver, M.D.

INTRODUCTION

Low-back pain is one of the major contributing factors of long term disability and loss of earning capacity in all industrialized societies. Disorders of the lower back rank second only to upper respiratory tract infections as a cause of loss of time from work. Backache is as old as mankind, or at least as old as mankind's first attempts to stand on his own two feet. Low-back pain, regardless of age or cause, plagues almost all of us at one time or another in either an acute or chronic phase. It could be said that this is the price paid for walking on our two hind legs. It has been estimated that almost 95 percent of the population will experience low-back pain during adult life. Over 200,000 laminectomies are performed annually in the United States, with reports of successful outcomes ranging from 40 percent to 96 percent, and patients with low-back pain of over six months duration represent a major segment of the permanently disabled.

Despite the frequency with which these complaints are encountered, the causes, preventions, definition of syndromes, and therapeutic programs associated with them remain highly problematic and controversial. Innumerable patients jump from one physician to another, seeking explanations for their subjective complaints and definitive treatment for their sometimes intractable enervating pain. The physician who treats low-back pain is faced with a great challenge, and one that is sometimes an enigma. Historical interview, physical examination, roentgenographic studies, laboratory analysis, and special studies—as we will discuss in this chapter—all help delineate the differential diagnosis and pathophysiological abnormalities of the lumbar spine. The etiological and psychosocial factors that often play an important part in our use of the musculoskeletal system, as well as the causes of low-back pain, will also be discussed.

Because spinal disorders produce such varying clinical pictures, there is a continuing effort to explain the mechanisms of pain. Human beings have suffered from back pain for thousands of years. Descriptions of various kinds of back pain can be found in numerous examples in the ancient literature. It is mentioned in the *Bible*, and Hippocrates, who lived in 400 B.C., spoke of sciatica. In some of Shakespeare's plays, the characters suffered from "lumbago."

Backache actually comes in two forms—acute and chronic. The majority of physicians usually see either one or the other, and both are characterized by varying degrees of pain and disability. The patient suffering from acute back pain often needs to go no further than the first physician he visits; the chronic back pain patient, on the other hand, usually ends up in the orthopaedist's office. Although backache is common, one can never underestimate the fact that an acute episode is a real emergency to the patient who is suffering. When the patient first comes to the physician, he is in pain and cannot move as freely or as fully as usual, whether due to spasm or to fear of increasing the pain. He may not know what's ailing him, but the chances are strong that he will suspect the very worst. Like all common maladies, backache has always been surrounded by a wealth of popular myths and misconceptions.

HISTORICAL REVIEW

Low-back pain and associated sciatica, formerly a syndrome of unknown etiology, has aroused the interest of medical research workers for almost two centuries. In this complex area of musculoskeletal disease, each and every generation of investigators has added a wealth of knowledge to our understanding and treatment of low-back pain, sciatica, and associated problems. The first to describe sciatica as a disease was Cotunnius (1764) who described three types of the disease: mainly, arthritic sciatica, in which pain was limited to the hip joint; nervous posterior and anterior sciatica, in which pain was confined to the posterior and anterior parts, respectively, of the leg; and muscular atrophy with associated symptoms of neuritis, including edema of the nerve sheath and consequent compression of the nerve. In doing so, he drew attention to the neural origin of the disease, distinguishing it clearly from joint pain.

In 1864, Lasegue described what is now the well-known *straight-leg raising* test. In 1904, the Frenchmen Lortat-Jacob and Sabareanu showed that certain causes of sciatica had a segmentary distribution of sensory disturbance. They introduced the term "sciatique radiculaire," which gained a firm footing with the work of Dejerine in 1916. The etiology of sciatica has been the subject of much speculation, and while many cases of intraspinal disc herniation had been reported as early as the 1800s, it was not until 1934 that Mixter and Barr showed that root compression due to disc herniation in the lumbar region was the commonest cause of sciatica. A case reported by Key (1838) of intradisc herniation from the eleventh thoracic interspace was about a patient whose disease resulted in paraplegia and death. In 1858, Luschka presented two cases of intraspinal disc herniation and demonstrated their relationship to herniated nucleus pulposus. This herniation produced no symptoms, but Luschka claimed that if these formations had grown or enlarged, they could have caused pressure on the spinal cord or nerve roots. Luschka's observations, however, passed unnoticed or into oblivion because with advances in spinal surgery, these symptomatic disc herniations became accessible to operation, and they were then regarded as tumors of the intervertebral disc. They were usually classifed as chondroma or fibrochondroma of the disc itself.

The first to report a case of traumatic dislocation of an intervertebral disc was Kocher in 1896. A 26-year-old man had fallen from a height of 100 ft. in a standing position. At autopsy, the disc between L1 and L2 showed a large bulge, but no vertebral fracture was demonstrable. Kocher believed the change to be due to protrusion but not proliferation. In 1911, Goldthwait published a paper in which he tried to find a relationship between sciatica and lumbosacral anomalies. He soon discovered, however, that many patients with congenital anomalies did not have sciatica, even though spina bifida occulta, sacralization and/or lumbarization of the vertebral bodies was present. Goldthwait concluded that subluxation of the lumbosacral joints was the commonest cause of sciatica.

In 1927, Schmorl described "knorpelknotchen": ruptures of the nucleus pulposus into the spongiosa. Two years later, Schmorl and Andrae described also "hintere Knorpelknotchen": ruptures of the nucleus pulposus into the spinal canal. These changes, however, were not of clinical importance in their opinion. In 1932, Schmorl and Junghans assumed ruptures might cause compression of the spinal cord if the ruptures achieved considerable dimensions. Several authors felt an irritation of the musculature might be the primary disorder responsible for sciatica. In 1908, Petran suggested that the puriformis, because of its close relationship to the sciatic nerve, might be particularly capable of affecting pressure upon the nerve. In 1920, Helweg postulated that the pathological anatomical cause of the disease was myopathic, probably of ischemic origin and due to muscular hyperfunction.

The speculations on the etiology of sciatica also included the doctrine of "viscerosensory reflex," as postulated by MacKenzie in 1893. According to that theory, sciatic pain is a type of "referred pain" from pathological changes in various joints in the lumbosacral region, or from the surrounding joints.

In 1918, Sicard felt that the site of irritation of the roots is situated peripheral to the spinal ganglion and is due to changes in the intervertebral foramen, which, by pressure against the spinal nerve, gives rise to sciatica. He called this form of sciatica "sciatique funiculaire," and Roger (1930) not only felt this to be the commonest form of sciatica, but further discovered that the changes in the intervertebral foramen were of rheumatic origin.

In 1925, Danforth and Wilson claimed, on the basis of a clinical and anatomical investigation, that sciatica pain is a symptom of injury to the lower lumbar region, commonly localized to the junction between L5 and the sacrum, and that the L5 root is the one primarily involved. After Mixter and Barr's 1934 renowned work had been published, many other series of operated disc herniations were ultimately reported in the literature. Love and Walsh in 1940 reported on over 500 cases and stated that 96 percent of the disc herniations were situated in the lower lumbar region. Naffziger and co-workers showed in 1938 that the ligamentus flavum might also be the cause of nerve root compression. This was a view shared by other neurosurgeons, specifically Barr and Malmros. According to Barr and Mixter in 1941, it was extremely difficult to ascertain preoperatively the level of disc herniation with certainty. No method for this was available at that time.

A great deal of medical research has been performed to help devise a reliable clinical method for localization of disc herniation. Today, we have numerous studies available to help us ascertain the level of intervertebral involvement, but it was the excellent work of Norlen in 1944 that first cleared the problems of discovering the location of the "compression syndrome" at any particular lumbar vertebrae and/or nerve root.

Surgical technique and methods have been devised mainly along the lines laid down by Mixter and Barr in the United States, and by Love and his associates—several excellent vertebral spine surgeons (Friberg, Olivecrona, Malmros, Sjoqvist and Hirsch) from the Scandinavian countries.

The possibility of outlining the spinal canal and its contents radiologically was suggested by Dandy in 1919, when he first described the air encephalography. He noted that the spinal cord would be outlined, and he predicted the use of this technique for the demonstration of spinal tumors. However, it was Jacobaens who performed the first myelogram in July 1919. He published his results in three cases in 1921, using air as a contrast medium. The use of contrast substance other than air began in 1922, when Secard and Forestier, who had been treating sciatica by the sacral injection of LIPIODOL, introduced a small quantity accidentally into the subarachnoid space. No one sued, and the potential value of this method for the demonstration of spinal space occupying lesions was realized at once. Although LIPIODOL gained widespread use in myelography, some of its properties were not altogether satisfactory. Pantopaque, introduced by Ramsey, French and Strain in 1944, proved more stable and cohesive and less opaque to x-rays, thus allowing a greater radiopacity of shadows on x-ray film. Soon thereafter, it replaced LIPIODOL in the United States. Amapaque and Isovue are now currently utilized in place of iodinated compounds.

In 1791, Galvani, in reporting his experiments with neuromuscular preparation of frog legs, demonstrated the two fundamental electrical properties of muscles: one, that muscle contracts when electrically stimulated and two, electrical current is produced during muscular contraction. The functional activity of a single motor unit was first recorded by Denny-Brown in 1929 and independently by Adrian and Bronk in the same year. However, Schiff, in 1851, was the first to observe fibrillation in the denervated muscle of a dog's tongue, five days after the hypoglossal nerve had been cut. He concluded that the oscillation (fibrillation) he observed in the denervated muscle was due to muscular activity and to the degeneration of the nerve. He noted that fibrillation ceased as the muscle atrophied, and that it also ceased when nerve regeneration took place.

Further work was done on fibrillation and denervation by Brown in 1937 and Denny-Brown and Pennybacker in 1938. They stated that the unit of action in fibrillation appeared to be from a single muscle fiber. Weddell, Finestein, and Pattle in 1943 and 1944 reported on the clinical application of electromyography (EMG). They noted fibrillation began 18–21 days after denervation. So, EMG has progressed with the transition from visual observation to the more accurate method of electrically recording fibrillation and denervation action potential. The EMG is now accepted as a definite adjunct to clinical medicine in neurology, orthopedics, and neurosurgery.

A presentation of this material would not be complete without giving consideration to the methods of diagnostic disc puncture and discography. A comparison of discography and diagnostic disc puncture with electromyography and myelography will not be included in this article.

Discography was first described in 1950 by Lindblom, a radiologist from Stockholm, Sweden. Lindblom conceived a method of demonstrating the nucleus pulposus roentgenographically by direct puncture of the disc through the spinal canal by injecting contrast material with a long, fine needle. In 1950, he reported on 38 patients who had had 52 lumbar discs injected for analysis. By 1962, Collis and Gardner claimed superiority for the method of lumbar myelography and detection of lumbar disc disease when they published their findings for over 1,000 cases. In 1948, Carl Hirsch published a paper on diagnostic disc puncture, postulating that rupture of the annulus fibrosis weakens the posterior border of the lower lumbar disc, thereby reducing the protection against mechanical strain. He felt it was justifiable to wonder whether an experimental increase in pressure within the disc would elicit lumbar pain. From a theoretical standpoint one can imagine a weakened posterior barrier, such as the posterior longitudinal ligament and/or annulus fibrosis, can allow for an increased deformity of the disc, with protrusion to occur in certain positions. This deformity could readily cause irritation of the posterior longitudinal ligament or annulus fibrosis, and be the etiology of some lumbar pain. Carl Hirsch studied the reactions of patients to stimulation and pressure on the posterior border of the lower lumbar disc and to an increase of intradiscal pressure by the injection of normal saline. Further, he studied the effect of lumbar pain of the injection of small quantities of local anesthetic into the intervertebral space. In all his cases, pain was produced from one or both of the lowest lumbar discs. In such cases where pain was produced from two discs, the patient could distinguish the different levels in the lumbar spine. In those cases in whom the puncture or movements of the needle increased the actual low-back pain, .5 cc of 1/10th percent Novocain had been utilized, for injection purposes. The increased pressure from the injection of Novocain was accompanied by temporary increase in the patient's pain. However, after two or three minutes the pain disappeared completely. The amount of anesthetic used was too little for the effect of anesthesia of the epidural tissue or nerve root to be permanent. When insertion of the needle did not cause pain, normal saline was injected under pressure. In some discs, the injection of saline produced little or no reaction; in others, up to 2 cc could be injected, and pain was sometimes produced when the pressure in the syringe was increased. When it was released, the patient's lumbago or subjective complaints of pain were relieved. Usually the patient was worse after the saline, but after some hours his original condition was restored.

Many investigators and vertebral spine surgeons have endorsed discography and disc injection methods as a successor to myelography in this country. However, many still feel it is another adjunct in the detection of discogenic disc disease rather than a replacement of myelography.

ANATOMY OF THE INTERVERTEBRAL DISC

Nucleus Pulposus

The intervertebral disc is the fibrocartilaginous complex that forms the articulation between bodies of the vertebrae. It provides a very strong union to allow the degree of intervertebral motion necessary for effective muscular action and the protective alignment of the spinal canal. Each intervertebral disc consists of two components: the internal hydrodynamic mass, the *nucleus pulposus* and its fibrous container, the *annulus fibrosus*. The nucleus pulposus is a remnant of the embryonic *notochordal* tissue. It is composed of loose, delicate fibrous strands imbedded in a gelatinous matrix. There is no definite structural interface between the nucleus pulposus and the annulus fibrosus. The composition of the two tissues blends together imperceptibly. The essential function of the nucleus is to resist and redistribute compulsive forces within the spine.

Annulus Fibrosus

The annulus fibrosus (A.F.) is a concentric series of fibrous lamellae encasing the nucleus and tieing the vertebral bodies strongly together. One of the major functions of the annulus is to withstand the tension from all the stresses placed upon the vertebral column.

Anterior Longitudinal Ligament

The anterior longitudinal ligament (A.L.L.) is a strong band of fibers that extends along the ventral surface of the spine from the skull to the sacrum. It is narrowest in the upper cervical region, where it is attached to the atlas and axis. It widens as it descends the column to the lower lumbar region. Most of the anterolateral surfaces of the vertebral bodies and discs are covered before it blends into the presacral fibers.

Posterior Longitudinal Ligament

The posterior longitudinal ligament (P.L.L.) extends from the skull to the sacrum. Being within the vertebral canal, its central fiber bundles must diminish in breadth as the size of the spinal column increases.

Sinuvertebral Nerve

The sinuvertebral nerve, a recurrent branch of each spinal nerve, is reflected back through the intervertebral foramen to supply fibers to the articular connective tissue, periosteum, meninges, and vascular structures associated with the vertebral canal. The nerve originates just distal to the dorsal root ganglion, where its frequent union with a branch from the ramus communicans reveals its dual spinal and autonomic composition. The sinuvertebral nerve passes through the superior part of the intervertebral foramen, usually between the dorsolateral surface of the vertebral body and its respective spinal nerve roots. Curving upward around the base of the pedicle, it divides into a superior and inferior branch on approaching the posterior longitudinal ligament. Numerous filaments are distributed throughout the course of the nerve to the periosteum, the posterior longitudinal ligament, and dura, and the epidural vessels. The nucleus pulposus has no sensory nerve supply, and the annulus fibrosus is innervated in its superficial layers only where it is most contiguous with longitudinal ligaments that also have a sensory supply.

HISTORY

Pain is subjective in nature. Subjective complaint is the patient's concept of what he is feeling, or experiencing. Detailed elucidation of its onset, character, distribution, and variation hopefully will give valuable insight into the underlying etiology. Very broadly, the different types of pain concerned may be defined as local, referred segmental, radicular, ischemic, and referred to the lower extremities as well as the lower-back area. Rarely is adequate information volunteered by the patient. Direct questioning of the patient is very important. An accurate description of the pain is of diagnostic importance

Some important questions to ask of a patient during the historical interview are as follows:

1. When did the pain start?
2. How did the pain start?
3. Locate the pain. Does it stay well localized? Where does it go? Up your back? Down your back? Into your legs?

4. Is it aching? Is it cramplike? Is it shooting in nature? Is it electrical in nature? Is it sharp and stabbing? Is it constant? Does it come and go (intermittent)?
5. What makes the pain worse? Standing? Walking? Sitting? Running? Jumping? Movements such as Valsalva maneuvers? Sneezing? Coughing? Having normal defecation? Or even micturition?
6. What makes the pain better? Rest? Positional changes? Medications? Heat therapy? Ice therapy? Hot tub baths or showers?
7. Is the pain more severe in the back or in the leg? Did it start in the leg and go to your back? Did it start in your back and go to your leg? Is it only in your back or only in your leg? Do you have loss of bowel or bladder control? Does coughing or sneezing cause you to lose water or soil your pants? Are you noticing any numbness or funny feelings or paresthesias in your back or legs? Are you weak or limping? Can you walk?

Through the detailed questions and answers that are supplied by the patients, the history can give great insight into the etiological background of the low-back pain. Correlations between pain and the structure of origin can help the clinician make a diagnosis. Pain usually arising in bone is of mild to moderate severity. Its distribution is local and its characteristics are usually constant with relief of pain at rest. Periosteal pain is usually of a more severe nature, with a local distribution constant in nature, making relief from it through rest rare. Disc pain ranges from mild to severe and is local in distribution; its characteristics vary with activity, and relief from pain is often obtained with rest. Spinal ligament pain is moderate in severity, its distribution is local or referred segmentally, its characteristics vary with activity and position, and relief with rest is usual. The pain severity of synovial joints is moderate. Pain is local and referred segmentally as far as distribution is concerned and varies with activity and position. Relief is usually attained through rest. Nerve root pain ranges in severity from minimal to excruciating, its distribution is radicular in nature, its characteristics vary with activity or position, and relief through rest is usual. Muscle shows its pain severity to be mild to moderate. The distribution of muscle pain is ischemic in nature, and it occurs only as a result of activity or positional change. Relief with rest can almost always be expected.

Low-back pain (a vague term) is a symptom, not a disease. The pathological cause of the symptom is most often to be found in the back itself, but it may also be discovered outside of the musculoskeletal system. One must, therefore, look at the genito-urinary, gastro-intestinal, or vascular system, as well as evaluating the musculoskeletal system. The back itself is subject to many disease processes; therefore, the differential diagnosis of low-back pain is variable.

The majority of patients (80 to 90 percent) with low-back pain fall into three specific categories: (1) acute and chronic lumbodorsal, musculotendinous sprain-strain complex; (2) degenerative arthritis of either the vertebral disc and/or apophyseal facet joints (These first two conditions are usually intermittently related rather than distinct, separate entities, although one may proceed the other as discogenic disc disease and/or facet degenerative osteoarthritic phenomena); (3) herniated nucleus pulposus, which can occur with or without nerve root impingement.

There are other causes of low-back pain which will be delineated in the course of this chapter.

ETIOLOGICAL FACTORS TO BE CONSIDERED IN THE DIFFERENTIAL DIAGNOSIS OF LOW-BACK PAIN

I. Mechanical

Mechanical factors are twofold, in that they may be related either to trauma or to a deformity. Regarding the trauma aspect of low-back pain, a soft-tissue injury resulting in a sprain-strain complex reveals that either the musculotendinous unit or the lumbodorsal ligamentous structures are stretched beyond their physiological limits. This is either caused by a sudden twisting, turning, bending, sneezing, coughing, or heavy lifting. If the acute episode has not been resolved within a period of approximately 6–8 weeks, and if it persists, it may very well become chronic if not treated successfully in an expeditious fashion. The sprain-strain complex usually causes moderately severe to excruciating pain with referred components, marked paravertebral spasm, and loss of range of motion of the lumbar spine. Positive, straight leg-raising will be associated in an ipsilateral and/or contralateral fashion. No focal motor nor sensory deprivation will be identified. Sitting, standing, walking, bending, and sleeping at night will be exceedingly difficult for the patient. Treatment consists of rest, analgesics, non-steroidal antiinflammatory drugs, avoidance of heat therapeutic modalities and use of cryotherapy, along with other specific physical therapy modalities.

The specific physical therapy modalities that may be utilized are electrical stimulation, laser therapy and, when the patient is symptom-free, a rehabilitative program to restore the strength and flexibility to the lumbodorsal and abdominal musculature. Ice is the best form of physical therapy to utilize for acute problems of the lumbar spine.

The bony structures can also be injured during a traumatic episode. Fracture of the vertebral body, as in a fall from a height with a compression fracture, or twisting torque mechanism of injury with fracture of the transverse spinous processes, all can cause severe excruciating pain with paravertebral spasm and loss of range of motion. Occasionally, one will see an acute pars intra-articularis defect in a young adolescent gymnast or other athlete, who will have an acute spondylolysis secondary to trauma, which oftentimes is not associated with a spondylolisthesis. Such fractures are usually related to the hyperflexion and/or hyperextension mechanism of injuries. These injuries can be with or without forced torque injury due to rotational aspects. Examples are seat-belt injuries, or falls from heights that are associated with other injuries.

Another aspect of the mechanical relates to deformities. Certain deformities are congenitally acquired. For example, there is spina bifida occulta, facet tropism asymmetry, and transitional vertebrae, where one has lumbarization of the sacral vertebra or sacralization of the last lumbar vertebra, along with scoliosis from a congenital hemivertebra. A spondylolysis with or without a spondylolisthesis, congenitally due to an elongated pars intra-articularis, has also been identified. Acquired deformities usually consist of spondylolysis, with or without associated spondylolisthesis, accentuated lordosis, or epiphyseal disorders predominantly related to Scheuermann's disease. Spondylolysis may not be symptomatic. Spondylolisthesis oftentimes will be symptomatic in the athletic individual, as well as in the patient doing heavy manual labor. There is no documented proof that spina bifida occulta, facet tropism or transitional vertebra are causative factors in low-back pain problems.

II. Degenerative Diseases

Degenerative diseases can occur involving either the disc, the synovial joint, or the arterial vasculature of the lower aorta limb vessels. The degenerative diseases that involve the disc consist of discogenic disc disease and osteoarthritis. Obviously, this is in an older age group than that of the young athletes in which the mechanical problems occur. These patients are, as a rule, 40 to 80 years of age. Symptoms will vary with activity and tend to be more referred in pain patterns than radicular. Often, local low-back pain without referral to the lower extremities is commonplace, especially at the beginning of the specific problem. If the patient develops severe enough degenerative osteoarthritis, where there is narrowing and/or encroachment of either the dura and its neural contents—or of the spinal nerve in the neural foramen—radicular symptoms can ensue. Verbeist described the syndrome of intermittent claudication of neural spinal origin due to vertebral spinal stenosis that is secondary to degenerative osteoarthritic phenomena of the disc and/or neural foraminal areas anatomically. This radicular type of pain is the result.

The herniated nucleus pulposus is by far one of the more prevalent forms of low-back pain. There are two types of herniated nucleus pulposi. One is contained within the annulus fibrosis, the other is noncontained, extruded beyond the annulus fibrosis and the posterior longitudinal ligament. Ninety percent of the herniated nucleus pulposi occur at L4–5 and L5-S1. The other 10 percent occur at L3–4. There are very specific signs and symptoms for the differential diagnosis at L3–4, L4–5 and L5-S1. The clinical features of a herniated nucleus pulposus at L3–4 disc will involve the 4th lumbar nerve root. The pain distribution will be in the lower back, hip, posterolateral thigh and the anterior leg down to the toe. Numbness will be in the anteromedial thigh and knee. Weakness may or may not be present in the quadricep mechanism, and atrophy may or may not occur circumferentially in the quadriceps mechanism. One reflex that will be diminished will be the knee jerk. A herniated nucleus pulposus at L4–5 involving the 5th lumbar nerve root will show a pain distribution pattern over the sacro-iliac joint, hip, and lateral thigh and leg. Numbness will be present in the web space between the first and second toes in the foot and over the proximal lateral aspect of the leg. Weakness in the dorsiflexion of the great toe and foot, especially the anterior tibialis, with difficulty walking on the heels and the potential for foot drop, may occur. Atrophy will be minor, although there may be some circumferential calf atrophy.

Reflexes show that changes are usually uncommon. However, an absent or diminished posterior tibial reflex may occur. The herniated nucleus pulposus at L5-S1 disc, involving the first sacral nerve root, will show a pain distribution over the sacro-iliac joint, hip, and posterolateral thigh and leg down to the heel. Numbness will be present over the posterolateral proximal back of the calf and the lateral heel, foot and toe, specifically the little toe. Weakness will be on plantar flexion of the foot and great toe, specifically the gastroc-soleus and flexor hallucis longus, and there will be difficulty walking on the toes. Atropy will be specifically in the calf because of the gastrocnemius and soleus. The ankle jerk reflex will either be diminished or absent altogether. A massive midline protrusion either at L4–5 and/or L5-S1 will show a pain distribution in the lower back, thighs, legs, and/or perineum, depending on the level of the lesion. Often, it will be bilateral rather than unilateral in pain distribution. The numbness is variable, to the thighs, legs, feet, and/or perineum, and may be bilateral more often than unilateral. Weakness is variable, with paralysis or paresis of the legs and/or bowel, with either bowel and/or bladder incontinence. This is obviously an acute cauda equina syndrome and therefore a surgical emergency. Atrophy may be extensive if left unattended. Reflexes show ankle jerk to be diminished or absent bilaterally.

Synovial joints, specifically the facet joints, can undergo facet impingement phenomena in which the lining membrane will be pinched or locked during flexion, extension and/or rotation. The patient will experience local pain in the lower back, an occasional referred pain, but, more importantly, there will be pain on hyperextension. This is the so-called facet phenomena and facet impingement syndrome. Facet degenerative osteoarthritic phenomena can also occur, and this is almost concomitant with an associated discogenic disc disease and/or osteoarthritic phenomena of the disc space. A settling phenomena puts abnormal biomechanical pressure and increased load forces on the facet joint, wearing out the facet joint and causing synovitis and synovial effusion of the facet joint, resulting in pain and discomfort. Paravertebral spasm ensues, with loss of range of motion, localized low-back pain, and occasional referred pain, but no radicular pain. Radicular pain can occur on rare occasions if facet hypertrophy becomes so great that the nerve root is impinged as it enters the neural foraminal canal. Other degenerative processes are those processes that occur in the abdominal aortic vasulature. Specifically, abdominal aortic aneurysm or iliac artery thrombosis. This pain creates claudication type symptomatology, with deficient pulses and other appropriate objective findings consistent with venous and/or vascular arterial insufficiency. Often, this is unilateral, but may very well be bilateral with white, pale, cold skin, and absent pulses, specifically in the posterior popliteal artery, posterior tibial artery, and dorsal pedal artery.

III. Inflammatory

Inflammatory diseases that can affect the lumbar spine are those that are infectious in nature. An acute pyogenic infection usually related to a Staphylococcus aureus coagulase positive organism will result in pain that is severe and excruciating. The patient will experience fever and chills, and chronic, dull low-back pain with or without referred pain may be the common subjective complaint. X-rays will show disc-space narrowing and/or an associated vertebral body osteomyelytic defect. The diagnosis is almost entirely dependent upon Craig needle biopsy, and obtaining the appropriate cultures to identify the organism. Definitive treatment follows, with the appropriate antibiotics administered intravenously. Many times the patient's history will reveal long-term substance abuse, heroin or, more recently, cocaine. Chronic pyogenic infection, such as that related to tuberculosis or, in the southwest, coccidioidomycosis, is not infrequent. Again, biopsy with Craig needle, with appropriate cultures and sensitivities, is usually the definitive means of diagnosis. Chronic pyogenic infections will often show a protracted history and weight reduction, with waxing and waning or exacerbation and aggravation of the symptomatology. X-rays of the area, with or without bone-scan technique, will often help to localize the specific anatomical area in the lower lumbar spine.

Acute pyogenic infections usually involve blood borne from a primary source in some other part of the body. The portal of entry is usually the respiratory tract in younger patients, and staphylococci are the most common pathogens. In older patients, the genitro-urinary tract is often the source of infection, especially after manipulative urological procedures. In these patients, the pathogen is more likely to be a gram negative rod. In rare instances, patients develop a disc-space infection postoperatively, following lumbar laminectomy and diskectomy. Chronic infections of the spine can be readily caused by mycobacteria organisms or brucella. Complaints of back pain in the chronic infections are accompanied by such symptoms as weakness, weight loss, night sweats, afternoon fever, protective listing, and scoliosis secondary to paravertebral spasm and loss of appetite.

Various noninfective processes will also cause low-back pain. The more common tends to be ankylosing spondylitis. The so-called Marie-Strumpell's disease is common in the lower back, will start specifically in the sacro-iliac joints. Chest expansion will be limited, and pain is well localized initially to the sacroiliac area and can be associated with paravertebral spasm and loss of range of motion and function of the lumbar spine. Uncommonly, rheumatoid arthritis will affect the lower back. However, other seronegative arthropathies such as Reiter's syndrome or psoriatic arthropathy can affect the lower back. Clinical historical interview and appropriate laboratory testing can give great insight into this particular problem. Pain tends to be well localized and referred to the lower extremities on occasion. The normal pattern tends to be morning stiffness that improves throughout the day, but gets progressively worse as the evening wears on. In the morning, it may take the patient anywhere from 45 minutes to an hour and a half after bathing and having breakfast before he or she can function. Treatment is, obviously, predominantly medical.

IV. Metabolic

There are various nutritional causes of low-back pain. Two specific causes are those related to osteoporosis and/or osteomalacia. Osteoporosis has a primary and/or secondary etiology. The primary causes of osteoporosis are a deficiency in metabolism of the aging male or female; congenital osteogenesis imperfecta, which is rare; estrogen deficiency, most commonly occurring in the post menopausal state naturally and/or induced, which is the most common cause of compression fractures in the elderly female group; or testosterone deficiency such as that related to Klinefelter's syndrome, hypogonadism, or castration secondary to tumor. Historical interview will give detailed information as to the specific etiology and whether or not this is associated with a compression fracture. Very often a patient will present with subjective complaints suggestive of a compression fracture and the examiner should be aware that these fractures can often be missed in early routine lumbar spine roentgenograms. If the patient's complaints persist, a bone scan, or technetium phosphate studies, will usually pick up these early micro fractures. Often compression fractures will be multiple and severely painful.

Secondary osteoporosis due to excessive catabolism can result from an excess of glucocorticoid steroids, as you would find in Cushing's syndrome. Prolonged immobilization due to illness or fracture treatment, as well as hyperthyroidism, are additional causes of secondary osteoporosis. Other associated causes are dietary in nature, for example, abnormalities stemming from the depletion of protein, calcium, or vitamin C. Achlorhydria, multiple myeloma, chronic leukemia, long-standing diabetes mellitus with ketoacidosis, liver cirrhosis, and acromegaly can also be causative factors. Why this happens is not explained, except on the basis of an excessive catabolism and an imbalance of hormonal factors.

Endocrinological aspects of secondary osteoporosis are those related to such problems as hyperparathyroidism or hypothyroidism, while steroid-induced osteoporosis with compression fractures is usually associated with steroid treatment of chronic obstructive pulmonary disease and other pulmonary abnormalities, as well as Cushing's disease and Paget's disease.

V. Neoplastic

Specific neoplastic problems can occur in the spinal column. Although not frequent in origin, benign tumors such as osteoblastoma, osteoid osteoma, aneurysmal bone cyst, and giant cell tumor—hemangioma—can occur in the bony structures of the posterior elements of the vertebral body, causing pain and discomfort, paravertebral spasm, and loss of range of motion. Hemangioma and osteoid osteoma tend to be more frequent tumors than the others. Treatment is by surgical excision when necessary and/or appropriate, with rehabilitation following surgery. Osteoid osteoma pain will often be relieved by aspirin and be more painful at night.

Secondary metastic lesions referable to primary tumors in the prostrate, breast, kidney, lung, thyroid and/or gastro-intestinal system will often cause excruciating night pain, weight-reduction anemia, paravertebral spasm, and loss of range of motion. The patient will often present several months to even years after the primary cancer has been treated. The metastatic lesion is found on either routine films or bone-scanning technique. Biopsy with a Craig needle for confirmation is helpful, and looking for estrogen receptor sites and drawing upon other special studies may be appropriate. Treatment is chemotherapeutic or radiologic, with or without surgical extirpation as necessary and/or appropriate. Benign tumors can occur that involve the meninges or nerve roots. These are usually meningomas or neurolemmomas. These are both very rare and can be treated successfully by surgical removal.

VI. Referred Pain Extrinsic

There are numerous aspects of pain that can be referred to the lumbosacral spine and cause paravertebral spasm and loss of range of motion. I refer to this as secondary low-back pain syndrome. Our colleagues in the obstetrics and gynecological field can see this in pregnancy, endometriosis, or with pelvic tumor such as uterine fibroids. Occasionally, pelvic inflammatory disease will cause low-back pain retroperitoneally.

Other aspects of peritoneal pain that can be observed by internists or nephrologists and gynecologists are renal tumor, hypernephroma, renal calculi, acute and chronic pyelonephritis, kidney infarcts, and prostatic disease, be it infectious or otherwise. Occasionally, low-back pain will result from gastro-intestinal diseases such as posterior penetrating ulcer, duodenal and/or gastric, with or without perforation; and pancreatitis, acute or chronic, with or without pseudocyst or tumor. Often, pancreatic carcinoma will present as low-back pain and the etiology be overlooked. Patients with carcinoma will present with low-back pain: the workup is negative, yet the patient still has severe, excruciating low-back pain, marked paravertebral spasm, and loss of range of motion. This pain tends to be moroe localized on the left side of the back and flank than on the right. Neurological findings are totally absent, and the examiner should be suspicious of carcinoma, especially when looking at an older patient presenting with this type of pain-pattern distribution. Unfortunately, it is often the case, that by the time the diagnosis is made, the patient has already suffered the pancreatic carcinoma and ultimate metastases, and usually succumbs within three to six months. In such cases, treatment is all too frequently ineffectual, as well as devastating to both the patient and his or her family. Occasionally, although rarely, patients with acute and/or chronic cholecystitis, with or without associated cholelithiasis, can suffer low-back pain.

More frequently, patients with sacro-iliac disease related to either trauma or infection—be it inflammatory, pyogenic, or noninflammatory, such as an ankylosing spondylitis—will present with low-back pain. A good historical interview and clinical examination with a positive Gaenslen's maneuver will show the patient's pain is related to the sacro-iliac joint. On rare occasion, degenerative osteoarthritis of the hip will cause retrograde pain to the back, specifically because of an antalgic gait and abnormal biomechanics.

A point needs to be made at this time referable to low-back pain and hip disease. Many patients will have discogenic disc disease, facet degenerative osteoarthritic phenomena or degenerative osteoarthritis of the lumbar spine. Occasionally, this will be associated with concomitant sacro-iliac disease or hip degenerative osteoarthritis. When a patient has back disease and hip disease, they are abnormally symbiotically related. One or both must be treated. The patient has to make the definitive decision as to which is the more tolerable to live with. Many times a patient who presents with concomitant disease will require total joint replacement for the hip disease; this will allow the patient to walk without an antalgic gait, giving increased range of motion, and thus relieve the biomechanical stress and forced strains placed upon the lumbar spine. It also allows conservative treatment to ensue for the lumbar spine in the usual methodical fashion. On rare occasions, due to embarrassment of neurological structures, prior to relieving the degenerative osteoarthritis phenomena of the hip, there might be required decompressive laminectomy, and/or foramintomy—as described in the literature by Verbiest, with regard to abnormalities and problems of the lumbar spine—in order that it may function even though the degenerative osteoarthritis phenomena of the hip has caused antalgic gait, loss of range of motion, and functional embarrassment of the hip joint. This is well delineated in the orthopedic literature, as well as in the experiences of Sir John Charnley at the hip center in Wrightington, England.

VII. Psychogenic Problems

Those patients who fall into the psychosomatic realm of unknown etiology, who might have conversion hysteria or acute hysterical reaction or even malingering at a conscious or subconscious level in order to gain some form of compensation, need to be evaluated just as meticulously, if not more so, than other patients. The physician in particular needs to be aware of the so-called Baron von Munchausen's syndrome. Patients with the syndrome show up in emergency rooms with severe excruciating low-back pain with a classic history for acute herniated disc, but against a background of few, if any, documented physical findings. Thus, the subjective complaints are totally out of proportion to the objective evidence. More importantly, the patient demands high-dose narcotics, intravenously, and intramuscularly as well as orally, almost every hour on the hour around the clock.

This syndrome is commonplace throughout the country. The medical literature is replete with cases of it, as well as of examples of patients in the United States working their way from one coast to another in anywhere from two days to two weeks, some of them even going so far as to allow surgical intervention in order that they might have the scar on their back confirming their need for narcotics. Psychiatric management, when appropriate, is advisable if the patient will comply.

On rare occasions, low-back pain will be observed in patients with diabetes mellitus, Charcot arthropathy secondary to disease entity such as syphilis, or alcoholism. Rare metal poisoning such as radium toxicity can also cause low-back pain.

Often, the historical interview can give the examiner a good idea of the differential diagnosis even before the physical examination. The experienced physician ask specific questions, check for appropriate responses, and have a high index of suspicion prior to examining the patient clinically.

VIII. Work-Related and Accidental Low-back Injuries

The physician who treats low-back disorders often finds himself faced with a patient who has pain all over—ill-defined pain—and who takes up a great deal of time both in the office and in the evening with phone calls. This is expressed as extraordinary pain, with subjective complaints not substantiated by objective findings, and appears as a persistent if not a chronic problem. In such cases, the physician who fails to recognize the anxious, apprehensive, or potentially hysterical patient does both the patient and himself a great disservice. Such a patient may exaggerate the story of a motor vehicle mishap or the amount of weight lifted at the time of injury, as well as other etiological aspects surrounding the traumatic insult and ultimate embarrassment, and sometimes the physician may fail to recognize the supra tentorial problems and need for definitive counselling, psychological and/or psychiatric.

Meeting with the family and/or employer is often important. The man who was at 18 capable of doing heavy manual labor, but who at age 50 is not, simply due to the normal aging process, is not therefore entitled to have his company pay for him to take it easy. Workman compensation injuries and the industrial laws in each state will vary and, thus, problems arising in the management of given patients in each state will vary. Conservative care must be the hallmark, if not the sine qua non of industrial injuries and workman compensation claims. However, nothing replaces good historical interview, physical examination, and proper diagnostic techniques. If a patient does, indeed, have a specific problem, i.e., herniated nucleus pulposus, and conservative management fails surgical intervention may become necessary. However, the patient, as well as the employer and the industrial insurance carrier, need to be made aware of the fact that the patient has had a specific job-related problem, i.e., herniated disc and heavy manual labor, and that, although the patient may be capable of doing some sort of job of that nature, restrictions and/or weight limitations may need to be placed upon the patient during his or her remaining years of gainful employment. Often, insurance carriers will not help in the rehabilitation of the older employee, on the other hand, if the patient is under a certain age, they will help with his or her rehabilitation and return to gainful employment. This is a highly problematic and frustrating area for the patient, the physician, the employer, and the industrial insurance carrier, to say the least.

Patients involved in slips and falls in grocery stores, commercial establishments, or motor vehicle mishaps often find themselves in a situation similar to that of those with industrial injuries and workman compensation claims. Proper historical interview, physical examination, ancillary tests, and x-rays are mandatory. The appropriate diagnosis and subsequent treatment, with good communication between the physician and patient, are also mandatory. Patients should not be led to believe they will end up perfectly normal after an injury unless the soft tissue component is of a minor nature. When patients require operative intervention, as in cases of herniated pulposus, whether it be by Chymopapain technique or laminectomy and diskectomy with definitive rehabilitation, patients should be aware they will experience some form of discomfort in the lumbar spine area for the remainder of their lives. Although they regain a good, full, free range of motion and the ability to enjoy recreational activities such as golf, tennis, racquet sports, and jogging, they should expect some form of a partial permanent impairment—as covered in the American Medical Association Guidelines—to be a normal result of treatment. In cases involving litigation, both the plaintiff's attorney and the defendant's attorney need to be clearly apprised of this fact, so that all are aware of the potential residual effects of the injury and the subsequent treatment that may be necessary.

PHYSICAL EXAMINATION

Patients with low-back pain should be completely disrobed except for their immediate undergarments; on occasion, even removal of the undergarments may be beneficial. Observation from behind the patient standing erect allows one to evaluate the lumbodorsal musculature of the vertebral column. It also allows the examiner to see if there is a neck and flank asymmetry, with one shoulder sitting higher than the other, or if a scoliotic curvature or list can be noted. Such observations must be documented. Next, the patient is evaluated in the walking position to see if there is any list in gait or antalgic component. The patient should be able to walk heel/heel or toe/toe or heel/toe with normal toe push-off in the normal gait attitude. The antalgic component or weakness such as a drop foot must be documented.

Palpation of the lumbodorsal musculature reveals if tightness and/or spasm is present or absent. Occasionally, pain may be palpated over the posterosuperior iliac spines where the lumbodorsal musculature inserts, as well as at the posterior iliac crest where the gluteus maximum originates. This particular area of the posterior iliac crest is not uncommonly involved in traumatic myofascial fibrositic type reactions secondary to trauma. If spasm is present in a moderate to severe degree, then a scoliosis or curvature of the vertebral spine will be observed. Some scoliotic curves assume different forms, based upon the underlying etiology, and may be either away from, or toward the herniated nucleus pulposus, depending upon the pathological lesion, which can be either lateral to the root (tension on the root is reduced by bending the trunk away from the lesion) or medial to the root (tension on the root is reduced by bending the trunk toward the lesion).

The range of motion of the lumbosacral spine should be documented. Do the fingertips touch the floor? Is there pain throughout the planes of range of motion during forward flexion or at the extremes of forward flexion? Is there pain throughout the planes of range of motion of extension of the lumbar spine or at the extremes of the lumbar spine? In order to see if there is severe limitation of motion at any specific level within the vertebral column, location of the apex of the various motions is important. The lumbosacral spine is capable of flexion, extension, lateral flexion, and lateral rotation. The normal components of motion will be observed in asymptomatic patients who do not exhibit a lumbodorsal musculature spasm or tightness. The patients who present with spasm will reveal a diminished range of motion as well as a flattening or loss of the normal lordosis within the lumbosacral spine. Spasm within the lumbodorsal musculature may be of a primary or secondary nature, as alluded to earlier in this chapter. Documentation of tightness or spasm reveals only that it exists, and it is not indicative of the etiological mechanism of pain.

A meticulous orthopedic and neurological assessment should be performed during the examination in order to discover whether there is an absence and/or diminuation of reflexes or sensory signs. Abnormal pathological reflexes should so be noted. The straight leg-raising and Lasegue's tests are both of significance, with reproduction of pain similar to the patient's subjective complaints. The Bragard test (dorsiflexion of the foot after the leg has assumed straight leg-raising position) has some validity in that the sciatic nerve is further placed on stretch; this is also true of the popliteal compression test. The Naffziger test is similar to the Bragard test, but performed in the sitting position. The patient should have straight leg-raising test, or modification of the straight-leg-raising test, performed sitting and supine. Radicular pain similar to the patient's subjective complaints, and reproduced by any of the above mentioned straight leg-raising tests, is indicative of entrapment phenomena of the nerve root most likely due to herniated nucleus pulposus or neural foraminal encroachment, such as subarticular gutter stenosis or vertebral spinal stenosis. Neurological deficits or motor deficits imply that the etiological factors are vertebral spine in origin. The level of the vertebral spine depends upon the underlying patho-physiological abnormalities.

Patients who present with subjective complaints with regard to the genito-urinary tract, gastro-intestinal abnormalities, or the female reproductive organs should routinely have a pelvic bimanual examination performed as well as a rectal examination. Occasionally, adnexal and rectal masses will be responsible for low-back pain.

WORK-UP OF PATIENTS WITH LOW-BACK PAIN

The patient with low-back pain may be ill enough and suffering enough acute pain to require hospitalization. The usual studies done in the hospital—or in a hospital laboratory serving outpatients—will help elucidate the etiology of low-back pain. The following tests are felt to be of importance: a CBC and sedimentation rate, and acid phosphatase and KDA 20. On rare occasions, rheumatoid factor or serum protein electrophoresis, as well as an immunodiffusion assay test and HLAWB–27 studies should be obtained. A clean-catch midstream urinalysis for microscopic urinalysis, as well as culture and sensitivity, are also appropriate.

The routine x-rays of the lumbosacral spine should be obtained either in the office or the hospital. An anteroposterior view, a lateral view, both oblique views, a spot view of lumbosacral spine, and sacro-iliac joint views are routine in most facilities. X-ray may show a narrowing of the disc space, with degeneration within the apophyseal facet joints. Spondylosis and osteophyte formation may be noted. Spondylolysis, a defect of the pars intra-articularis with or without associated spondylolisthesis, may be readily apparent on just routine films. Other roentgenographic manifestation may reveal osteoporosis, compression fractures, metabolic bone disease, benign or malignant tumors, disc space infection, and osteomyelitis of the vertebral body.

Special roentgenograms will include lumbar discography, or myelography when indicated. Computerized axial tomography and magnetic resonance images may also be indicated for delineating etiological causes of low-back pain. Plain x-rays are the first line of thought. If the plain x-rays give information, then often one may not have to advance to the more special, highly expensive roentgenographic studies. More frequently than not, to be thorough in the delineation of lesions, advanced studies like computerized axial tomography, magnetic resonance imaging and subsequent myelographic studies, or even discography, will follow during the clinical evaluation of the patient's pain. When discography is called for, it can be done either with the saline or water acceptance technique, or with radiopaque material, to document the roentgenographic evaluation of the disc as described by Lindbloom in Sweden.

Numerous neurologists, neurosurgeons, and orthopedic surgeons rely on electromyographic interpretation, along with nerve conduction velocities of the lumbosacral spine and peripheral lower extremities. Often, the correlation between the EMG and myelogram leaves the clinician somewhat frustrated. It has been said that electromyography is only as good as the electromyographer. The same is true of the myelogram. In previous years lumbar myelography was performed using Pantopaque, an oil-based, iodinated, radiographic compound, which had to be retrieved after the procedure. This resulted in unnecessary pain and discomfort for the patient. With the introduction of water-soluble compounds which do not require retrieval, such as Amapaque and, more recently, Isovue, the myelogram now has fewer complications and side effects and is more readily accepted, with less fear and apprehension, by the patient. All in all, however, electromyographic interpretation, even in the best of hands, is only 80 percent efficient in evaluation, and lumbar myelography is only 85 percent efficient. There is about a 10 to 12 percent false positive aspect to lumbar myelography and a 5 to 6 percent false negative aspect. The etiology of these false positive and false negative aspects has yet to be elucidated in the medical literature.

Bone-scan techniques are of importance with enlargements or snap studies of the lumbar spine. They can pick up early compression fractures or early neoplastic metastatic lesions. The same is true when correlating bone-scan and computerized axial tomography or magnetic resonance imaging studies. When myelographic studies are performed, analysis of the spinal fluid is of tantamount importance. Culture and sensitivity, cell count, protein evaluation, and virology studies for syphilis as well as protein electrophoretic patterns may be appropriate to rule out demyelinating diseases such as multiple sclerosis.

Recently, thermography has elicited a great deal of interest with regard to the evaluation of the lumbar spine. Although controversy exists about the interpretation of thermograms, it would appear that there may be a role for thermography in this regard in the future. More importantly, if the patient has a reflex sympathetic dystrophy—the so-called "post causalgia syndrome" in the lower extremities—due to low-back pain factors, thermography may be more diagnostic of this particular problem. More work and research in this area, as well as further experience, will elucidate the significance and helpfulness of thermography.

There are several other studies in the interpretation and evaluation of low-back pain patients that may come into play. Often, patients who have had a lower-back injury—with subsequent diagnosis of and definitive treatment for herniated nucleus pulposus, and operative intervention—may end up with the so-called "failed lumbar laminectomy syndrome." Scar tissue and/or adhesions with and without any evidence of arachnoiditis may ensue. Patients have consistency in their complaints or do well for a short period of time, only to get progressively worse as time goes on. Many of them who have had previous laminectomy and diskectomy, with persistency of pain, may require nerve root injection studies, Pentothal pain study, or epidural venography study with an abdominal compression test to help elucidate the significance and persistency of their specific subjective complaints, with or without previous objective findings. Pentothal pain study is advised for the patient who has low-back pain with a positive straight-leg-raising test and a paucity, as a rule, of neurological sensory or motor deprivation evaluation. The straight leg-raising test is persistently causing the patient pain sitting and/or supine, with or without referred and/or radicular symptomatology, and subjective complaints will be out of proportion to the objective findings. With the patient asleep, the Pentothal pain study can elucidate as to whether the pain is organic and/or functional. Often, malingering can be documented, with the patient actually laughing and/or showing a perfectly normal examination. The reader is referred to the earlier Pentothal pain study article written by the author.

The epidural venography study tends to give good information in the virgin back; however, in the patient with failed lumbar laminectomy syndrome, it may not give as much information as may be desired, especially if the problem is at the same disc space level. Nerve root injection studies are of excellent benefit for a specific nerve root, and thus the reader is referred to the orthopedic literature for the benefits of this particular study.

Baseline blood studies such as CBC and sedimentation rate will show evidence of infection and/or anemia. High white-cell count with a shift to the left showing segmented neutrophilis is elucidated. Excessively elevated sedimentation rate is often found in disc space infection and/or vertebral osteomyelitis. Abnormalities in any of the 20 channel KDA studies is quite obvious. Hyperurecemia with or without an acute attack of gouty arthropathy of the lumbar sacral spine is easily delineated on the KDA 20, as well as from the historical interview. Kidney disease with abnormalities and elevations of BUN and creatinine, or any abnormal findings such as liver function test and alkaline phosphatase, will be delineated by KDA 20. Those patients who have prostatic metastatic disease will have an elevated acid phosphatase. Those patients who have seronegative arthropathy and/or connective tissue disorders will have abnormal findings in the serum protein electrophoresis, immunodiffusion assay test, or HLA WB 27 studies. Thus, laboratory studies are of benefit and can help in the differential diagnosis.

TREATMENT

The treatment of low-back pain is best approached by first making accurate and proper diagnosis. In general, patients with low-back pain diagnosed to have one of the three more common problems (acute and chronic lumbodorsal musculotendinous strain, degenerative arthritis of either the vertebral disc and/or apophyseal facet joints, or herniated nucleus pulposus) can be treated in a successful conservative fashion with bed rest for a minimum of five to ten days and a maximum of twenty one to twenty eight days. Bed rest may or may not be associated with pelvic or Buck's traction. If the patient is hospitalized, one reason for the traction may purely be to make sure he or she remains restfully in bed. Pelvic and/or Buck's traction has no beneficial effects biomechanically unless the weights on it exceed one-third of the patient's body weight. Thus, the efficacy of traction ofoten lies only in that it keeps the patient in bed for a prescribed period of time in order to place the lumbodorsal musculature, and other vertebral spine elements at rest and relaxation.

The position of the patient in bed is the so-called Gatch position. This is a combination of either the Williams or the semi-Fowler position. The waist is bent, the knees and hip are bent, and the legs are elevated.

The patient with low-back pain usually presents to the physician with severe pain, spasm, and loss of range of motion of the lumbosacral spine. Pain relief through appropriate analgesics can be of great benefit, regardless of the etiology. Non-narcotic analgesics can often be utilized to alleviate the patient's pain. Occasionally, narcotic analgesia is of benefit, either by intramuscular and/or oral administration. The decision to use these should be at the discretion of the treating physician, with a view to the patient's needs. I, myself, never use narcotic analgesics in or out of the hospital, favoring instead medications such as steroids: Medrol 4 mg, 1 q.i.d. for two days; 1 t.i.d. for 3 days; 1 b.i.d. for four days; and 1 every morning for four days. If I don't use a steroid and go instead to a nonsteroidal anti-inflammatory drug, I have found Naprosyn very beneficial to the patient with vertebral spine abnormalities. However, the clinician can use any of the excellent nonsteroidal anti-inflammatory drugs available, based upon the patient's needs.

This treatment can occur in or out of the hospital, as necessary. I use nonsteroidal anti-inflammatory drug to alleviate a patient's pain. It does this by acting at the primary focus of pathophysiological abnormality. On many occasions, I will utilize skeletal muscle relaxants with the nonsteroidal anti-inflammatory drug. The two best skeletal muscle relaxants are Flexeril, 10 mg at bedtime, and/or Valium, 5 mg in the morning and 10 at bedtime. Valium tends to be one of the finest skeletal muscle relaxants as well as having a tranquilizing effect upon patients extremely apprehensive and anxious over their acute low-back pain problem. Other muscle relaxants given orally are of little efficacy, in my opinion, primarily because the absorption rate is poor. The only other medications for skeletal muscle relaxation that I have been successful with have been intravenous Robaxin and/or intravenous Norflex. The efficacy of other medications, such as Robaxin, Norgesic, Parafon Forte, Soma Compound, or any of the various generic skeletal muscle relaxants, traditionally taken orally, has, in my opinion, been obscured by poorly documented double blind studies, and in my personal and professional experience I have found them to be of little benefit to the patient.

I would like to take this opportunity to condemn the utilization of heat therapeutic modalities, and to caution the reader to avoid all of them. I tell my patients unequivocably to avoid heat. No hot showers, no hot tub baths, no heating pads, no hot water bottles, no rubbing linaments, no BenGay, no analgesic balms. They are to unequivocably stay away from saunas, Jacuzzi, steam baths, or any other heat therapeutic modalities. In my experience, the patient's comfort while using the heat therapeutic modality lasts only a short period of time, usually 5, 10 or 15 minutes, only to be followed by excessive pain a half hour to one hour later. This is the direct result of heat application, which causes a deterioration in the condition of the lumbodorsal musculotendinous unit, increasing pain, spasm, tightness, and discomfort.

I recommend unequivocably, as does the orthopedic medical literature, cryotherapeutic modalities. Ice massage, ice packs, and avoidance of heat is of mandatory importance. The ice acts as a superficial analgesia and therapeutic treatment for the acute inflammation of the anatomical complex in the posterior elements of the vertebral spine and the lumbodorsal muscles. Ice is utilized both on an outpatient basis, in physical therapy departments, and in the hospital. Numerous forms of cold packs are available. Ice should never be applied directly to the skin except by a trained physical therapist. If the patients are utilizing ice and other cryotherapeutic modalities at home, they are cautioned to wring a hand towel or wash cloth under cold water, apply the towel or wash cloth to their back, and then place the ice over it, so the coolness can penetrate the cloth and act as a moist, cold compress to anesthetize the area and diminish swelling and pain by direct vasoconstriction. The reason for avoiding heat is that heat therapeutic modalities result in vasodilation and increase the blood supply and the inflammatory response.

On many occasions, patients will be started immediately on physiotherapy modalities. Often, low-dose ultrasound, ice massage, ice packs electrical stimulation, and possibly even laser therapy may be utilized in a physical therapy prescription for acute low-back pain syndrome. Careful reevaluation on an inpatient hospital basis day-to-day will delineate whether the patient is progressing favorably or not. Not infrequently, due to the socioeconomic problems that many people have in today's society, it may be advantageous for the orthopedic surgeon to seek a clinical psychological evaluation and obotain an MMPI test.

If patients are treated with the conservative mode of rest, cryotherapy and other physiotherapy modalities, and with the prescribed medications mentioned earlier in this article, there should be a relatively rapid response both from the patient's point of view and in terms of the clinical assessment by the physician.

The vast majority of patients will respond favorably to conservative nonoperative management of the lumbosacral spine. As delineated earlier, the proper clinical diagnosis will help in the response to the conservative care. Consultation, when deemed necessary, is of importance in assuring proper diagnosis and to confirm specific etiological factors. Those patients who have failed to resolve their symptoms after a reasonable period of nonoperative management should be considered for surgical intervention. The appropriate studies, consisting of a combination of any and all of the following, should be performed as an ancillary aid to the orthopedic and/or neurosurgical colleagues treating the patient, myelography, computerized axial tomography, magnetic resonance imaging, electromyographic and nerve conduction velocity studies, and possibly even discography. If the diagnosis is one of herniated nucleus pulposus, then the patient and physician need to evaluate the efficacy of Chymopapain. There are specific indications and contraindications for Chymopapain injection of a herniated nucleus pulposus. As a rule, however, those patients who are considered excellent candidates for laminectomy and diskectomy can readily be considered candidates for chemonucleolysis by the Chymopapain injection.

Contraindications for Chymopapain are as follows: (1) any patient having received Chymopapain previously; the reason for this being the potential for sensitization and possible allergic reaction; (2) patients having failed lumbar laminectomy syndrome without interval improvement of symptoms or findings, unless failed laminectomy is due to a missed herniated disc. It may be that the level is different and the patient may have had a herniated nucleus puposus at L4–5, and now has a herniated nucleus pulposus at L5-S1; L5-S1 can be injected. In the hands of the experienced vertebral spine surgeon, or a vertebral spine surgeon utilizing Chymopapain, the patient may want to have the Chymopapain and/or collagenase injection prior to another operation. This consideration is not to be entertained by the patient or the surgeon without a great deal of thought and informed consent. (3) A rapidly progressing neurological deficit. (4) A significant neurological deficit producing a severe bowel or bladder symptom complex. (5) Evidence of spinal cord tumor. (6) Serious concurrent illness. (7) History of allergy or hypersensitivity to papaya or papaya derivatives, beer, meat tenderizer. These patients need to be properly skin-tested with RAST testing. (8) No pregnant patients are candidates for the procedure. (9) Spinal stenosis or spondylolisthesis.

Relative contraindications in which one might consider not utilizing chemonucleolysis with Chymopapain: (1) Herniation of more than one disc, although in the hands of some people this is not a contraindication. However, utilization in such cases requires a great deal of experience on the part of the vertebral spine surgeon as well as the informed consent of the patient. (2) Severe degenerative disc disease at levels other than that to be injected. (3) Any third-party payment for back injury or similar circumstances or history of medical litigation. This includes motor vehicle mishaps, slips and falls in commercial establishments, and workman compensation industrial injuries. (4) Diabetes mellitus. The reason for this is that many diabetics have peripheral neuropathy and, although the patient may have herniated nucleus pulposus—and the symptomatology from the HNP will resolve along with some of the radicular component—the patient's peripheral neuropathy would as a rule be persistent, with the patient not getting the desired relief from pain or discomfort. (5) Evidence of impaired motivational characteristics, or a significant psychogenic component to the symptomatology.

I have had personal experience with approximately 110 patients with chemonucleolysis and Chymopapain injections. I have injected on approximately 8 patients two disc space levels. The majority have been for an isolated herniated nucleus pulposus, predominantly at either L4–5, L5-S1 or infrequently, at L3–4. The results have been very efficacious, though I have had 8 failures. In the 8 failures, 6 patients did well after laminectomy and diskectomy for an extruded fragment that was trapped in the neural foraminal canal. The other two cases were abysmal failures necessitating further surgery and stabilization, and to this date, these patients, both of whom are receiving workman compensation, still have chronic back problems. All told, however, in my experience, Chymopapain injection for chemonucleolysis has been an exceedingly beneficial and efficacious treatment modality for herniated nucleus pulposus.

For those patients who undergo laminectomy or laminotomy with diskectomy, the surgical technique will vary. However, the approach is basically the same, and the results are intended to eliminate pain by removing the pathological herniated nucleus pulposus and allow the patient to return to some form of functional capacity. Often, the patient will undergo decompressive laminectomy with disketomy and foraminotomy. The more severe the problems, the greater the intensity and magnitude of the surgical procedure.

The hallmark of postoperative management is to rehabilitate the lumbodorsal musculature once the wounds have healed. The rehabilitation period may require a minimum of 3 to 6 months and maximum of 6 to 12 months and will vary from patient to patient depending on age, sex, appropriate diagnosis, motivational factors, and concomitant illness.

In the operating room at the time of surgery, it has been this author's habit to document the level of the herniated nucleus pulposus by placing a #18-gauge spinal needle in the disc space and confirming the level with plain x-ray in the lateral projection of the lumbar spine. Thus, the clinical correlation and ancillary roentgenographic studies, along with findings observed at operation and documentation of the disc space level that one is performing a diskectomy on is not left to chance but is documented intra-operatively in the operating room. If a patient has a herniated nucleus pulposus at L4–5, and if the findings correlate subjectively and objectively, roentgenographically, myelographically and/or on computerized axial tomography, then the confirmation is correlated. At the time of surgery I approach the L4–5 space, place a needle in it, find the herniated nucleus pulposus with or without extruded fragment, take an x-ray and see that I am operating at the right disc space level. This is of great importance to me as the vertebral spine surgeon. It is my usual protocol to take the x-ray in the operating room. During the surgical procedure, it is routine for me to check up and down the canal and in the foramen; up, down and around in the axilla and shoulder of the root; and make sure no extruded fragments have been overlooked or missed.

In order to prevent scar tissue from occurring, it became my habit to use a ligamentum flavumotomy technique by which the ligamentum flavum was preserved, the herniated nucleus pulposus was removed, and the ligamentum flavum was utilized to cover the dura and the nerve root. In addition, a hemovac drain was used to drain any accumulation of blood and thus the potential for hemutoma or postoperative wound infection was also diminished. In the patient with failed lumbar laminectomy syndrome who has subsequently undergone operative intervention at the same level of cicatrix, recurrent herniated nucleus pulposus, or neural foraminal encroachment, a pedicle fat graft or free fat graft is done to help prevent scar tissue invasion. The reader is referred to the orthopedic literature for the ligamentum flavumotomy technique and the pedicle fat graft technique as described by this author.

It has not been the habit of this author to utilize lumbersacral spine fusion at the time of laminectomy and diskectomy. If an arthrodesis of the lumbosacral spine is necessary for mechanical reasons such as spondylolysis and/or spondylolisthesis or facet DJD phenomena, then fusion has been done in the posterolateral fashion utilizing Luque rod instrumentation and Wisconsin wires and bilateral posterolateral fusion at the appropriate levels. Surgical technique for this is well delineated in the orthopedic literature. Damage to the dura, whether to the nerve roots or to its spinal contents, is very demanding on the vertebral spine surgeon, and meticulous technique is adhered to during the operative procedure.

The author has had experience in a small number of cases with anterior interlumbar body spine fusion. The literature is replete with information, and Sir Harry Crock of Australia has devised specific instrumentation, as well as a technique, for this procedure. Although Crock testifies to excellent results, it has not been this author's experience that the results have been anything but poor to fair at best. Often, the patients end up with nonunion of the anterior interlumbar body spine fusion area and their problems persist. If done as a salvage operation, the procedure meets with failure. In addition, in the male patient, the complication of impotency and sexual dysfunction is a possiblity that needs to be discussed in detail prior to surgery. Although this author has not had any experience with posterior interlumbar body spine fusion, the technique developed by Cloward is one that should be condemned. While in Cloward's hands its results may be excellent, this has not been the experience of this author. Although I have not done one personally, I have seen innumerable patients that had posterior interlumbar body spine fusion—the so-called P.L.I.F. procedure performed by experienced neurosurgeons and orthopedic surgeons. These patients became visibly and demonstrably vertebral spine cripples, with tremendous problems of cicatrix, arachnoiditis, nonunion, neural element damage, in any combination. I would caution the reader to be exceedingly concerned when there is a recommendation that the experienced vertebral spine surgeon do a posterior interlumbar body spine fusion at the time of a simple laminectomy and diskectomy, or even when considering a salvage operation. Well-respected vertebral spine centers throughout the country have echoed this criticism of Cloward's technique.

With a proper diagnosis of the etiology for low-back pain having been made on behalf of a given patient, and the subsequent definitive successful treatment with conservative care having occurred, the patient can resume normal activities. However, as previously stated, in those patients where conservative care has failed and operative intervention is necessary, the patient has a choice between chemonucleolysis or laminectomy and diskectomy. It is this author's advice not to recommend laminectomy, diskectomy or arthrodesis at the time of disc excision. Sticking to the empirical evidence is to the patient's advantage, and if, indeed, he or she develops at some later date a biomechanical problem or other related problem that would require arthrodesis, then it should be done, with or without instrumentation such as Luque or Harrington rods. Patients should be informed that internal fixation devices such as screws, and Harrington and/or Luque rods with or without wires may need to be removed at some future date due to bodily reactions, or the loosening or breakage of relatively inert materials.

MEDICOLEGAL CONSIDERATIONS

One obvious problem in treating low-back pain is that the etiology of the back pain is difficult to demonstrate with any high degree of certainty or accuracy. Thus, treatment is often empirical with a prolonged course. Many physicians will become disheartened during the first few weeks of treatment; they may eventually come to look upon each new back pain victim as just "another crock to be evaluated."

Low-back pain is only a symptom, and one must search diligently to make a proper diagnosis. Thus, one of the medicolegal considerations in treating this condition is the possibility of incorrect diagnosis and/or incorrect evaluation of the studies necessary to making a proper diagnosis. The physician who orders electromyography studies needs to be aware that a number of anatomical and physiological factors are responsible for the deficiency of electromyography as a 100 percent accurate diagnosis tool for determining the level of nerve root compression or abnormality. One factor is variance in the normal anatomy of the nerve root, such as conjoined nerve roots. The second is that electromyography may be done too early, for example, before the first six weeks of nerve root compression. The third is that the disc, if herniated, can be a midline herniation or a far-lateral herniation in which subjective complaints with some objective findings may be present even though the root specifically involved may not be compressed, and the electromyography will be negative. Far-lateral herniation and midline herniation may not have enough specific root involvement to show up in electromyographic studies. In addition, sensory involvement will sometimes only be symptomatic; thus a mixed nerve as a peripheral nerve may have the herniation and compression on the sensory area and not the motor area, and failure to pick it up by electromyographic studies is not uncommon. They may also fail to strike the denervated muscle fibers, thus, the statement that the electromyographic studies are only as good as the electromyographer has been promulgated.

With regard to myelographic evaluations, I have already alluded to the frequent occurrence of false positive and false negative myelograms. There are also complications from myelography stemming from technical considerations, myelographic materials, and idiosyncratic reactions and interpretation by radiologists, whether they be trained in neural radiology or diagnostic radiology only. Failure to perform the study properly and/or failure to interpret the study properly obviously has medicolegal implications.

In view of neural radiology having become a distinct entity in the last five years, complete with advanced techniques consistent with computerized axial tomography and magnetic resonance imaging studies, it has been this author's experience that, if a myelogram is to be performed, I would like to have the computerized axial tomography done within the first four hours of completion of the myelographic evaluation of the lumbar spine. This then gives a myelographic enhanced computerized axial tomogoraphy, which is far more useful to the neuroradiologist, as well as to the experienced vertebral spine surgeon than just a myelogram. This is my recommended protocol for patient diagnostic evaluation.

Appropriate consultations with neurologists, neurosurgeons, and orthopedic surgeons for confirmation of level and/or diagnosis may be necessary, depending upon the community and environment of your particular circumstances and/or hospital atmosphere. Many insurance companies, specifically industrial carriers, mandate second opinions. I have for a long time personally recommended second opinions in a nonrelated specialty. I am an orthopedic surgeon, and I ask neurologists and neurosurgeons for clinical confirmation and opinions of my diagnosis and recommended treatment or therapeutic procedures. I am exceedingly conservative and, in cases where conservative care has failed and I must recommend surgical intervention, I usually draw upon a neurosurgeon or neurologist for clinical confirmation and evaluation of the patient. Only after the consultant confirms the diagnosis, states unequivocably that conservative care has been an absymal failure, and concurs in the advisability of surgical intervention, do I, with the approval of the patient and the patient's family, go ahead with an informed consent for the recommended treatment.

Following failure of both conservative care and operative intervention, before the patient is going to have a Chymopapain injection for chemonucleoysis purposes, he or she is shown a filmed lecture on Chymopapain pointing out the advantages and disadvantages, inherent risks, the potential allergic complications, etc., of such a measure. I see to it that, by seeing this movie, listening to their physician, reading medical literature and talking to other patients, these patients are sufficiently knowledgeable to decide whether by informed consent they wish to go ahead and have the chemonucleolysis procedure performed.

The same consideration is given to the patient who must decide whether to undergo laminectomy and diskectomy for herniated nucleus pulposus. The more information the physician can provide patients in order for them to make an appropriate decision, the better for all parties concerned. The medicolegal implications of this are obvious, to say the least.

At the time of surgery, the complications from Chymopapain are technical: incorrect placement of the needle, poor evaluation of discography studies by water or saline acceptance at the time of discography, failure to adhere to the meticulous technical protocol, and overutilization of the amount of Chymopapain. Thus, the complications and problems that can ensue are of major neurological embarrassment to the patient, and can sometimes lead to anaphylaxis, paralysis, and death. Again, the medicolegal implications are obvious.

The procedure of both laminectomy and diskectomy is fraught with numerous technical problems. One can miss a piece of disc fragment that is trapped out of sight and even the best surgeon searching most meticulously may not find the disc fragment, which will then come to cause recurrent problems for the patient at some point, whether sooner or later, after the operation. In addition, if an excessive amount of bleeding from epidural veins is present, and the vertebral spine surgeon does not have clear vision, one can damage the dura, the root, or both. The battered root syndrome is well delineated in the orthopedic literature. The patient at time of laminectomy and diskectomy can have the wrong disc space level operated on. This is not unheard of either in the orthopedic and neurosurgical literature or in various malpractice cases tried due to poor results in vertebral spine surgery. It thus behooves the experienced vertebral spine surgeon to make a proper diagnosis, select an appropriate form of treatment on behalf of his or her patient, and manage the technical procedure diligently, carefully, and meticulously, with proper planning preoperatively, intra-operatively, and postoperatively. The medicolegal considerations here are self-explanatory.

One of the technical complications of lumbar spine surgery documented in orthopedic literature is laceration of the abdominal vasculature, such as the abdominal aortic artery or iliac artery. Arterial damage is not such an infrequent occurrence and, if unrecognized, it can lead to demise of the patient. The reader is referred to the orthopedic literature for a discussion of this particular complication, the recognition of which is quite obvious in the intra-operative frame, since there is both excessive bleeding and compromise of the patient's vital signs. Emergency vascular surgery care is mandatory.

Postoperative management of the patient with lumbar spine surgery is anything but routine. Many patients after surgery on the lumbar spine develop reflex ileus, and keeping them NPO after surgery for a minimum of 12 and maximum of 48 hours may be appropriate. Within 24 to 48 hours, the hemovac drains are removed from the lumbar spine. The patients are up and sitting about within 24 to 48 hours and ambulating at 72 hours. The placement of high thromboembolic stockings is necessary. Watching patients closely for thrombophlebitis and any compromise in the lower extremities is important. My particular protocol tries to avoid anticoagulation drugs except when necessary and/or appropriate because of specific history or previous utilization. This is managed by an internist with mini-dose heparin until wound-healing is satisfactory and no compromise or potential for hematoma is present. When the patient is eating properly, eliminating satisfactorily with good bowel and bladder function, and showing no evidence of any wound problems discharge from the hospital and appropriate outpatient planning is mandated. Often, patients like to wear lumbosacral corset postoperatively for a short period of time. Those patients who have had arthrodesis performed wear a rigid high lumbosacral chairback brace, which is considered beneficial.

Problems that ensue postoperatively in patients include thrombophlebitis, pulmonary difficulties with atelectasis, fever and/or pneumonitis, and genitro-urinary tract infections dur to instrumentation of the bladder by Foley catheter. Thus, the patients need to be instructed postoperatively to watch for fever, chills, urgency, frequency, dysuria, or any increasing pain in the back or legs if surgery had resolved their previous back and leg pain.

In addition, patients are alerted to the fact that many medications can potentially cause allergic reactions or side effects. Counseling is given in regard to these medications at the time of the patient's discharge. If problems ensue, the patient should be directed to call the physician or his service immediately. The medicolegal implications of this are straightforward.

CONCLUSION

The methods of treatment for low-back pain are legion and usually depend upon the bias and experience of the vertebral spine surgeon or individual physician. Most low-back problems tend to be related to a strain-sprain complex that can be controlled by conservative treatment and cured with nonoperative measures. Other problems, such as disc disease, can similarly be treated conservatively and, if operative intervention is necessary after proper diagnosis, tend to usually respond favorably to either Chymopapain and/or laminectomy and diskectomy procedures.

Maintaining improvement and preventing recurrence are the objectives of treatment for low-back pain. Walking and swimming help to achieve these aims. Sports that require twisting and abrupt turning such as golf or tennis must be approached with caution, since the lumbar spine is quite vulnerable to such rapid movements. In any event, a cardinal rule for persons prone to low-back pain should be to avoid activities that push them beyond the physiological limits of their muscles, tendons, ligaments, or disc complex. The author has articulated an approach, considering both the anatomic and historical background, to the etiological significance of low-back pain. Also covered have been the differential diagnosis of low-back pain, as well as various studies used to arrive at the appropriate diagnosis, and the definitive forms of treatment for the condition, be they surgical or conservative. In addition, some medicolegal considerations and common pitfalls and complications attending the subject have been discussed. For more specific elucidation of the complex aspects of the lumbar spine, the reader is referred to the bibliography.

The author would like to take this opportunity to give his deepest and most sincere thanks and appreciation to Mary Lou Christensen, CMT, for typing and revising the manuscript, and to Shannon Hardy, R.N., and Margot N. Silver, clinical coordinator, for their editing of the manuscript.

REFERENCES

1. Abel, M. S. "Oblique motion studies and other non-myelographic roentgenographic criteria for the diagnosis of degenerative intervertebral disc." *American Journal of Surgery*, 99:717–26, 1960.

2. Abrams, H. L. "Skeletal metastases in carcinoma." *Radiology* 55:534–38, Oct, 1950.

3. Albbe, F. H. "Transplantation of a portion of the tibia into the spine for Pott's disease: A preliminary report." *JAMA*, 57:885–886, Sept, 1911.

4. Alexander, G. A. "Prolapsed intervertebral discs." *Edin. Med. J.* 54:14–29, 1947.

5. American Orthopedic Association Research Committee, Nachlas, I. W., Chairman, End-result of a study of the treatment of herniated nucleus pulposus by excision with fusion and without fusion, *J. Bone & Joint Surg.* 34A:981, 1952.

6. Anderson, G. W., and Alpers, B. J. "Retroperitoneal tumor as cause of low back and leg pain." *Neurology* 3:553–562, Aug, 1953.

7. Aranson, H. A., and Dunsmore, R. H. "Herniated upper lumbar discs," *J. Bone Jt. Surg.* 45-A:311–17, 1963.

8. Armstrong, J. R. "The causes of unsatisfactory results from the operative treatment of lumbar disc lesions." *J. Bone Jt. Surg.* 33B:31–35, Feb. 1951.

9. Armstrong, J. R. *Lumbar disc lesions*, 3rd ed, London: E & S Livingstone Ltd., 1965, 307.

10. Badgley, C. E. "The articular facets in relation to low-back pain and sciatic radiation." *J. Bone Jt. Surg.* 23:481–96, April, 1941.

11. Barr, J. S. "The operative management of low-back pain." *American Academy of Orthopaedic Surgeons Instructional Course Lectures*, vol. V, Ann Arbor: J. W. Edwards, 1948, 291.

12. ———. "Low-back and sciatic pain, the results of treatment. *J. Bone Jt. Surg.* 33A:633–49, July, 1951.

13. ———. "Sciatica caused by intervertebral disc lesions, *J. Bone Jt. Surg.* 19:323, 1937.

14. ———. "Ruptured intervertebral disc and sciatic pain, *J. Bone Jt. Surg.* 29:429–37, April, 1947.

15. Barr, J. S., Hampton, A. O., and Mixter, W. J. "Pain low in the back and 'sciatica' due to lesions of the intervertebral discs." *JAMA* 109:1265, 1937.

16. Barr, J. S., and Mixter, W. J. "Posterior protrusion of the lumbar intervertebral disc," *J. Bone Jt. Surg.* 23:444–456, 1961.

17. Begg, A. C. F. "Nuclear herniation of the intervertebral disc: Their radiological manifestations and significance." *J. Bone Jt. Surg.* 36B:180–93, May, 1954.

18. Begg. A. C. and Falconer, M. A.: "Plain radiology in intraspinal protrusion of lumbar intervertebral discs correlated with operative findings." *British Journal of Surgery*, 36:225–39, 1949.

19. Bhagwati, S. N., and Ginde, R. G. "Prolapsed lumbar intervertebral disc (A follow-up of 60 operated cases). "Neurol., India, 4:14–17, 1956.

20. Bick, Edgar M. "The osteohistology of the normal human vertebra," *Journal of Mount Sinai Hospital*, XIX 3, Sept/Oct., 1952.

21. Bobechko, W. P. "Autoimmune response to nucleus pulposus in the rabbit." *J. Bone Jt. Surg.*, 47B:574–580, Aug., 1965.

22. Bosworth, D. M. "Cases simulating posterior herniation of the nucleus pulposus of the intervertebral disc." *American Academy of Orthopaedic Surgeons Instructional Course Lectures*, vol. VIII, Ann Arbor: J. W. Edwards, 1951, 327.

23. ———. "Further notes on cases simulating posterior herniation of the nucleus pulposes of the intervertebral disc." *American Academy of Orthopaedic Surgeons Instructional Course Lectures*, vol. IX, Ann Arbor: J. W. Edwards, 1952, 71.

24. Bradford, F. K., and Spurling, R. G., *The Intervertebral Disc*, 2nd ed., Springfield, IL: Charles G. Thomas, 1947.

25. Brady, L. P., Parker, L. B., and Vaughen, J. "An evaluation of the electromyogram in the diagnosis of the lumbar disc lesion," *J. Bone Jt. Surg.*, 51A:539–47, 1969.

26. Brish, A., Lerner, M. A., and Braham, J. "Intermittent claudication from compression of cauda by a narrowed spinal canal." *J. Neurosurg.*, 21:207–211, March, 1964.

27. Bucy, P. C., Heimburger, R. F., and Oberhill, H. R. "Compression of the cervical spinal cord by herniated intervertebral discs." *J. Neurosurg.*, 5:471, 1948.

28. Bull, J. W. D. "Rupture of the intervertebral disc in the cervical region." *Proc. Roy. Soc. Med.*, 41:513, 1948.

29. Bull, J., and McKissock, W. *An Atlas of Positive Contrast Myelography*. New York and London: Grune and Stratton, 1962.

30. Caldwell, G. A., and Sheppard, B. "Criteria for spine fusion following removal of the protruded nucleus pulposus." *J. Bone Jt. Surg.*, 30A:971–80, Oct., 1948.

31. Campbell, Willis C. "Operative measures in the treatment of affections of the lumbosacral and sacro-iliac articulation." *Surg. Gyne. and Obst.*, 51:381, 1930.

32. Chandler, F. A. "Lesions of the isthmus of the lower lumbar vertebrae and their relation to spondylolisthesis." *S.G.O.*, 53:273, Sept., 1931.

33. Cloward, R. B. "The treatment of ruptured lumbar intervertebral disc by vertebral body fusion, III Method of use of banked bone." *Ann. Surg.*, 136:987, 1952.

34. ———. "The treatment of ruptured lumbar intervertebral discs by vertebral body fusion, I. Indication, operative technique, after care." *J. Neurosurg.*, 10:154, 1953.

35. Cloward, R. B. and Buzaid, L. L. "Discography: technique, indications and evaluation of the normal and abnormal intervertebral disc." *Am. J. Roentgenol.*, 68:552, 1952.

36. Colonna, P., and Friedenberg, Z. B. "The disc syndrome: results of conservative care of patients with positive myelograms." *J. Bone Jt. Surg.*, 31A:614–18, July, 1949.

37. Compere, E. L. "Spinal fusion following removal of intervertebral disc." *South. M.J.*, 39:301, 1946.

38. ———. "Origin, anatomy, physiology and pathology of the intervertebral disc." *American Academy of Orthopaedic Surgeons Instructional Course Lectures*, vol. XVIII, Ann Arbor: J. W. Edwards, 1961, 15.

39. Compere, E. L., and Keyes, D. C. "Roentgenologic studies of intervertebral discs, discussion of embryologic, anatomy, physiology, clinical and experimental pathology." *American Journal of Roentgenology*, 29:774, 1933.

40. Cramer, F., and McGowan, T. J. "Role of nucleus pulposus in pathogenesis of so-called "recoil" injuries of the spinal cord." *Surg. Gyne. and Obst.*, 79:516, 1944.

41. Crue, B. L., Pudenz, R. H., and Sheldon, C. H. "Observation of the value of clinical electromyography." *J. Bone Jt. Surg.* 39A:492–500, June, 1957.

42. Dandy, W. E. "Concealed ruptured intervertebral discs: plea for elimination of contrast medium in diagnosis." *JAMA*, 117:821, 1941.

43. Duncan, W. R., and Hoem, T. I. "A new approach to the intervertebral disc." *S.G.O.* 75:257–67, Aug., 1942.

44. Elsberg, C. A. "Experiences in spinal surgery: observations upon 60 laminectomies for spinal disease. *Surg. Gyne. and Obst.*, 16:117, 1913.

45. Epstein, J. A., Epstein, B. S., and Lavine, L. S. "Nerve root compression associated with narrowing of the lumbar spinal canal." *J. Neurol. Neurosurg. Psychiat.*, 25:165–176, May, 1962.

46. Epstein, J. A. "Diagnosis and treatment of painful neurological disorders caused by spondylosis of the lumbar spine." *J. Neurosurg.*, 17:991–1001, Nov., 1960.

47. Eyre-Brook, A. L. "A study of late results from disc operations." *Brit. J. Surg.*, 39:289–96, 1952.

48. Falconer, M. A., McGeorge, M., Begg, A. C. "Observations on the cause and mechanism of symptom production in sciatica and low-back pain." *J. Neurol. Neurosurg. Psychiat.*, 11:13–26, 1948.

49. Ferguson, A. B. "Roentgenograph of the lumbosacral area." *American Academy of Orthopaedic Surgeons Instructional Course Lectures*, vol. IV, Ann Arbor: J. W. Edwards, 1947, 89.

50. Ferguson, A. B. "The clinical and roentgenographic interpretation of lumbosacral anomalies." *Radiology*, 22:548, May, 1934.

51. Ford, L. T., and Key, J. A. "An evaluation of myelography in the diagnosis of intervertebral disc lesions in the low back." *J. Bone Jt. Surg.*, 32A:257–66, April, 1950.

52. Ford, L. T., Ramsey, R. H., Holt, E. P., and Kay, J. A. "Analysis of 100 consecutive lumbar myelograms followed by disc operation for relief of low-back pain and sciatica." *Surgery*, 32:961–66, 1952.

53. Friberg, S. "Low-back and sciatic pain caused by intervertebral disc herniation." *Acta Chirgica Scandinavia*, 85: Supplement 64, 1–114, 1941.

54. Friberg, S., and Hirsch, C. "Anatomical and clinical studies on lumbar disc degeneration." *Acta Orthopaedica Scandinavia*, XIX:222–42, 1949.

55. Friedman, J. and Goldner, M. A. "Discography in evaluation of lumbar disc lesions." *Radiology*, 65:653, 1955.

56. Gewanther, A. P., Mitchell, N., and Angrist, A. "Latent Primary Carcinoma." *Arch. Path.*, 35:66:84, Jan., 1943.

57. Ghormley, R. K. "Diagnosis of lame backs." *American Academy of Orthopaedic Surgeons Instructional Course Lectures*, vol. I, Ann Arbor: J. W. Edward, 1943, 106.

58. ———. The problem of multiple operations on the back." *American Academy of Orthopaedic Surgeons Instructional Course Lectures*, vol. XIV, Ann Arbor: J. W. Edwards, 1957, 56.

59. ———. "Low back-pain with special reference to the articular facets." *JAMA*, 101:1773–77, 1933.

60. ———. "An etiologic study of backache and sciatica pain." Proceedings Staff Meetings of the Mayo Clinic, 26:457, 1951.

61. Gillespie, H. W. "Radiological diagnosis of lumbar intervertebral disc lesions: A report of 160 cases." *Brit. J. Radiol.*, 19:420–28, 1946.

62. Goldthwait, J. E. "The lumbosacral articulation: Explanation of many cases of "lumbago," "sciatica," and "paraplegia." *Boston Med. Surg. J.*, 164:365–72, 1911.

63. ———. Backache, *New England J. Med.* 209:722, 1933.

64. ———. "Low back lesions." *J. Bone Jt. Surg.*, 19:810, 1937.

65. Grant, F. C. "Operative results in intervertebral discs." *J. Neurosurg.*, 1:332, 1944.

66. Grant, F. C. "Operative results in intervertebral discs." *Ann. Surg.*, 124:1066, 1946.

67. Gurdjian, E. S., and Webster, J. E. "Lumbar herniations of the nucleus pulposus." *Am. J. Surg.*, 76:235, 1948.

68. Gurdjian, E. S., Webster, J. E., Ostrowski, A. Z., Hardy, W. G., Lindmer, D. W., and Thomas, M. "Herniated intervertebral disc analysis of 1176 operated cases." *Journal of Trauma*, 10158–76, 1961.

69. Haggart, G. E. Discussion of Spurling, R. G., Mayfield, F. H. and Rogers, J. B. "Hypertrophy of the ligamenta flava as a cause of low back pain." *JAMA* 109:928, 1937.

70. Hallock, H. "Low-back lesions-anatomical considerations." *American Academy of Orthopaedic Surgeons Instructional Course Lectures*, vol. IV, Ann Arbor: J. W. Edwards, 1947, 87.

71. Hansen, H. J. "Disc degeneration in dogs." *Acta Orthopaedica Scandinavia*, 20:280–93, 1950.

72. Harbison, S. P. "Major vascular complications of intervertebral disc surgery." *Ann. Surg.*, 140:342, 1954.

73. Harmon, P. H. "Indications for spinal fusion in lumbar discopathy, instability, and arthrosis." *Clinical Orthopedics*, 34:73–107.

74. Harmon, P. H. "Anterior disc excision and fusion for intervertebral disc syndrome in the low lumbar spine." *Clinical Orthopedics*, 26:107, 1963.

75. Harmon, P. H., and Morton, S. A. "Correlation of multiple objective diagnostic methods in lower lumbar disc disease." *Clinical Orthopedics*, 28:132, 1963.

76. Harris, R. I. "Spondylolisthesis." *Ann. Roy. Coll. Surgeons, England*, 8:259, 1951.

77. Harris, R. I., and MacNab, I. "Structural changes in lumbar intervertebral discs: Their relationship to low-back pain and sciatica," *J. Bone Jt. Surg.*, 36B:304–322, May, 1954.

78. Hauser, E. "The treatment of low-back pain due to functional decompensation." *American Academy of Orthopaedic Surgeons Instructional Course Lectures*, vol. II, Ann Arbor: J. W. Edwards, 1944, 435.

79. Hawk, W. A. "Spinal compression caused by ecchondrosis of the intervertebral fibrocartilage, with a review of the recent literature." *Brain*, 139:204, 1936.

80. Hirsch, C. "Efficiency of surgery in low-back disorders." *J. Bone Jt. Surg.* 47A:991–1004, July, 1965.

81. Hirsch, C. "Mechanical response in normal and degenerated lumbar discs." *J. Bone Jt. Surg.* 38A:242–43, Jan., 1956.

82. Hirsch, C. "Studies on the pathology of low-back pain." *J. Bone Jt. Surg.* 41B:237–43, May, 1959.

83. Hirsch, C. "An attempt to diagnose the level of a disc lesion clinically by disc puncture." *Acta Ortho. Scandinavia*, 18:132, 1948.

84. Hirsch, C., and Shajewicz, F. "The studies on structural changes in the fibrous annulus." *Acta. Ortho. Scandinavia*, 22:146, 1952.

85. Holscher, E. C. "Vascular complications of disc surgery." *J. Bone Jt. Surg.*, 30A:968, 1948.

86. Holt, E. P. "The question of lumbar discography." *J. Bone Jt Surg.*, 50A:720–26, 1968.

87. Hubeny, J. J., and Mass, M. "Roentgenologic Aspects of Metastases." *Radiology*, 35:315–21, Sept., 1940.

88. Hunt, A. B. "Backache of gynecologic origin." Proceedings of Staff Meeting of the Mayo Clinic, 26:480, 1951.

89. Hurteau, E. F., Baird, W. C., and Sinclair, E. "Arachnoiditis following the use of iodized oil." *J. Bone Jt. Surg.*, 36A:393, 1954.

90. Inman, V. T., Saunders, J. B., de C. M. "Referred pain from skeletal structures." *J. Nerv. Ment. Dis.* 99:660–667, May, 1944.

91. Jaslow, I. A. "Intercorporal bone graft in spinal fusion after disc removal." *Surg. Gyne. & Obst.*, 82:215, 1946.

92. Josey, A. I., and Murphey, F. "Ruptured intervertebral disc simulating angina pectoris." *JAMA*, 131:581, 1946.

93. Kahn, E. A. "The role of the dentate ligaments in spinal cord compression and the syndrome of lateral sclerosis." *J. Neurosurg.*, 4:191, 1947.

94. Kambia, P. S., Smith, J. M., and Hoerner, E. F. "Myelography and electromyography in the diagnosis of herniated intervertebral disc." *JAMA*, 181:472–75, Aug., 1962.

95. Kaplan, L., and Kennedy, F. "The effect of head posture on the manometrics of the cerebrospinal fluid in cervical lesions: A new diagnostic test " *Brain*, 73:337, 1950.

96. Keegan, J. J. "Dermatome hypalgesia associated with herniation of intervertebral disc." *Arch. Neurol. & Psychiat.*, 50:67, 1943.

97. Kelley, J. H., Voris, D. C., Svien, H. J., and Ghormley, R. K. "Multiple operations for protruded lumbar intervertebral disc." Proceedings of Staff Meeting of the Mayo Clinic, 29:546, 1954.

98. Kellgren, J. H. "On the distribution of pain arising from deep somatic structures with charts of segmental pain areas." *Clin. Sci.*, 4:35, 1939.

99. Kallio, K. E. "Experiences with the problem of low-back pain and sciatica." *American Academy of Orthopaedic Surgeons Instructional Course Lectures*, vol. XIV, Ann Arbor: J. W. Edwards, 1957, 23.

100. Knutsson, B. "Comparative value of electromyography, myelography, and clinical neurologic examination in the diagnosis of lumbar root compression syndrome." *Acta Ortho. Scandinavia*, Supplement 49:1–135, 1961.

101. Key, J. A. "The intervertebral disc: anatomy, physiology and pathology." *American Academy of Orthopaedic Surgeons Instructional Course Lectures*, vol. VI, Ann Arbor: J. W. Edwards, 1949, 27.

102. ———. "The conservative treatment of low-back pain and sciatica." *American Academy of Orthopaedic Surgeons Instructional Course Lectures*, vol. VI, Ann Arbor: J. W. Edwards, 1949, 39.

103. ———. "Anatomy, physiology, and pathology. *Academy of Orthopaedic Surgeons Instructional Course Lectures*, vol. XI, Ann Arbor: J. W. Edwards, 1954, 101.

104. ———. "Intervertebral disclesions in children and adolescents, *J. Bone Jt. Surg.*, 32A:97, 1950.

105. Keyes, D. C., and Compere, E. L. "The normal and pathological physiology of the nucleus pulposus of the intervertebral disc: An anatomical, clinical, and experimental study." *J. Bone Jt. Surg.*, 14:897, 1932.

106. Kuhns, J. G. "Medical causes of backache." *American Academy of Orthopaedic Surgeons Instructional Course Lectures*, vol. V, Ann Arbor: J. W. Edwards, 1948, 280.

107. Lansche, W. E., and Ford, L. T. "Correlation of the myelographic clinical and operative findings in the lumbar disc lesion." *J. Bone Jt. Surg.*, 42A:193–206, March, 1960.

108. Leader, S. A., and Rossel, M. J. "Value of pantopaque myelography in the diagnosis of herniated nucleus pulposus in the lumbosacral spine." *American Journal of Roentgenology*, 69:231–241, Feb., 1953.

109. Light, S. "*Electrodiagnosis and electromyography.*" New Haven: Elizabeth Licht, 1956.

110. Lindblom, K. "Diagnostic puncture of intervertebral discs in sciatica." *Acta Ortho. Scandinavia*, 17:231, 1948.

111. Lindblom, K., Rexed, B. "Spinal nerve injury in dorsolateral protrusions of lumbar discs." *J. Neurosurg.*, vol. 5, 5, 413–32, 1948.

112. Lindblom, K. "Experimental ruptures of intervertebral discs in rat's tails." *J. Bone Jt. Surg.*, 34A:no. 1, 123–28, Jan., 1952.

113. Lindblom, K. "Technique and results of diagnostic disc puncture and injection (discography) in the lumbar region." *Acta Ortho. Scandinavia*, vol. XX, 315–26, 1951.

114. ———. "Discography of dissecting transosseous rupture of disc in lumbar region." *Acta Rad.*, 36:12, 1951.

115. ———. "Technique and results in myelography and disc punture." *Acta Rad.*, vol. XXXIV, 321–30, Oct/Nov., 1950.

116. Logue, V. "Thoracic intervertebral disc prolapse with spinal cord compression." *J. Neurol., Neurosurg. & Psychiat.*, 15:227, 1952.

117. Love, J. G. "Special nerve root retractor used in removing protruded intervertebral discs." Proceeding of Staff Meeting at the Mayo Clinic, 12:393, 1937.

118. Love, J. G., and Kiefer, E. J. "Root pain and paraplegia due to protrusions of thoracic intervertebral discs." *J. Neurosurg.*, 15:62, 1950.

119. Love, J. G., and Rivers, M. H. "Spinal cord tumors simulating protruded intervertebral discs, *JAMA*, 179:878–81, March, 1962.

120. Love, J. G., Walsh, M. M. "Intraspinal protrusion of the intervertebral disc." *Arch. Surg.* 40:454–84, 1940.

121. Low-Back Symposium. *J. Iowa M. Soc.*, 51:629, 1961.

122. Luck, J. V. "Discogenic syndromes - factors in differential diagnosis." *American Academy of Orthopaedic Surgeons Instructional Course Lectures*, vol. XVIII, St. Louis: C. V. Mosby Co., 1961, 35.

123. Marinacci, A. A. *Clinical electromyography: A brief review of the electrophysiology of the motor unit and its application to the diagnosis of myopathies*. Los Angeles: San Lucal Press, 1955.

124. Massie, W. K. "Comparative study of spinal fusion by the combined interbody and posterior element method with the Hibb posterior element fusion and with H-graft modifications, *J. Bone Jt. Surg.*, 41A:1358, 1959.

125. McK., Craig, W., et al. "Intraspinal lesions masquerading as protruded lumbar intervertebral discs." *JAMA*, 149:250–53, May, 1952.

126. McRae, B. L. "Asymptomatic intervertebral disc protrusions." *Acta Rad.*, 46:9–27, Sept., 1955.

127. Mendelsohn, R. A., and Sela, A. "Electromyography in herniated lumbar disc." *Arch. Neur. & Psychiat.*, 79:142–145, Feb., 1958.

128. Meyerding, H. W. "Low-backache and sciatic pain associated with spondylolisthesis and protruded intervertebral disc: incidence, significance, and treatment" (symposium). *J. Bone Jt. Surg.* 23:461, 1941.

129. Mixter, W. J., and Barr, J. S. "Rupture of the intervertebral disc with involvement of spinal canal." *New Eng. J. Med.* 211:210–215, Aug., 1934.

130. Muller, R. "Protrusion of thoracic intervertebral disc with compression of the spinal cord." *Acta Med. Scandanavia*, 139:99, 1950.

131. Murphey, F., Pascucci, L. M., Meade, W. H., and Van Zwaluwenburg, B. R. "Myelography in patients with ruptured cervical intervertebral discs." *Am. J. Roentg.*, 56:27, 1946.

132. Nachlas, W. "End-result of a study of the treatment of herniated nucleus pulposus by excision with and without fusion." *J. Bone Jt. Surg.*, 34A:981–988, Oct., 1952.

133. Naffziger, H. C., Inman V., Saunders, J. B., and deC. M. "Lesions of the intervertebral disc and ligamenta flava: clinical and anatomical studies." *Surg. Gyne. & Obst.* 66:288, 1938.

134. Newman, P. H. "The etiology of spondylolisthesis." *J. Bone Jt. Surg.*, 45B:39, 1963.

135. Ober, F. R. "Back strain and sciatica." *JAMA* 104:1580, May, 1935.

136. O'Connell, J. E. "Protrusion of the lumbar intervertebral disc: A clinical review based on 500 cases treated by excision." *J. Bone Jt. Surg.*, 33B:8–30, Feb., 1951.

137. Odell, R. T., and Key, J. A. "Results of the operative treatment of ruptured intervertebral discs." *American Academy of Orthopaedic Surgeons Instructional Course Lectures*, vol. VI, Ann Arbor: J. W. Edwards, 1949, 43.

138. Oppenheimer, A., and Turner, E. L. "Discogenic disease of the cervical spine with segmental neuritis." *Am. J. Roentg.* 37:484, 1937.

139. Owen, W. B. "Spinal fusion (Higgs') operation for Pott's disease: exhibition of patient." *Kentucky Med. J.*, 27:122–24, March, 1929.

140. Paulson, S., Sylvan, B., Hirsch, C., and Snellman, O. "Biophysical and physiological investigations on cartilage and other mesenchymal tissues. III the diffusion rate of various substances in normal bovine nucleus pulposus." *Biochimica et Biophysica Acta*, 7:207–213, 1951.

141. Percy, O. "Contrast media examination of the intervertebral disc of the lower lumbar spine." *Acta Ortho. Scandinavia*, 20:327–34, 1950.

142. Phalen, G. S. "Backache caused by vascular disease." *Clin. Ortho.*, vol. 5, 149–54.

143. Poppen, J. *The Herniated Intervertebral Disc*. Phila.: Surgical Practice of the Lahey Clinic, W. B. Saunders Co., 1951, 777–83.

144. Puchel, J. "Wassergehalt normaler and degenerieter, Zwischenwirbelscheiben." *Beitr. Path. Anat.*, 84:123–130, Feb., 1930.

145. Putti, V. "New conception in pathogenesis of sciatic pain." *Lancet*, 2:53–60, July, 1927.

146. Raaf, J. "Some observations regarding 905 patients operated on for protruded lumbar intervertebral disc." *Am. J. Surg.*, 97:388–99, 1959.

147. Ramsey, R. H. "Conservative treatment." *American Academy of Orthopaedic Surgeons Instructional Course Lectures*, vol. XI, Ann Arbor: J. W. Edwards, 1954, 118.

148. Ray, S. S. "Lesions simulating disc protrusion." *American Academy of Orthopaedic Surgeons Instructional Course Lectures*, vol. VII, Ann Arbor: J. W. Edwards, 1950, 244.

149. Reynolds, F. C., McGinnis, A. E., and Morgan, H. C. "Surgery in the treatment of low-back pain and sciatic: A follow-up study." *J. Bone Jt. Surg.*, 41A:223–35, March, 1959.

150. Rinonapoli, E. "L'Ernia del disco Intervertebrale nell eta senile." *G. Geront*, 8:449–56, April, 1960.

151. Rolfe, P. G. "Innervation of annulus fibrosus and posterior longitudinal ligament: fourth and fifth lumbar level." *Arch. Neurol & Psychiat.*, 44:100, 1940.

152. Ross, P., and Jelsma, F. "Postoperative analysis of 366 consecutive cases of herniated intervertebral disc." *Am. J. of Surg.*, 84:657–62, 1952.

153. Sarin, M. G., and Chandy, J. "A follow-up study of lumbar intervertebral disc protrusion." *Neurology, India*, 7:71–73, 1959.

154. Schmorl, G. "Zur pathologischen Anatomic der Lendenbandscheiben." *Klin. Wsch.*, 11:1369–71, August, 1932.

155. Schmorl, G., and Junghanns, H. *Archiv. und Atlas der normalen und pathologischen Anatomie in typischen Rontgenbildern*. Leipzig: Georg Thieme, 1932.

156. Schneider, C. C. "Diagnosis, treatment and rehabilitation of the industrial low-back cripple." *American Academy of Orthopaedic Surgeons Instructional Course Lectures*, vol. XVI, Ann Arbor: J. W. Edwards, 1959, 173.

157. Scoville, W. B., Whitcomb, B. B., and McLaurin, R. "The cervical ruptured disc; report of 115 operative cases." *Tr. Am. Neurol A.*, 76th Ann. Meet. 222, 1951.

158. Seeley, S. F., Hughes, C. W., and Jahnke, E. J., Jr. "Major vessel damage in lumbar disc operation." *Surgery*, 35:421, 1954.

159. Semmes, R. E. "Diagnosis of ruptured intervertebral disc without contrast myelography and comment upon recent experience with modified hemilaminectomy for their removal." *Yale J. Biol. & Med.*, 11:433, 1939.

160. Semmes, R. E., and Murphey, F. "The syndrome of unilateral rupture of the sixth cervical intervertebral disc with compression of seventh cervical root: report of four cases with symptoms simulating coronary disease." *JAMA*, 121:1209, 1943.

161. Semmes, R. E., and Schultz, E. C. "Personal communication, 1955.

162. Shapiro, R. "Myelography." in *Chicago Year Book Med.*, 1962.

163. Shaw, E. G., and Taylor, G. "The results of lumbosacral fusion for low-back pain." *J. Bone Jt. Surg.* 38B:485–97, March, 1956.

164. Shea, P. A., Woods, W. W., and Werden, D. H. "Electromhography in the diagnosis of nerve root compression." *Arch. Neurol. & Psychiat.*, 64:93–104, July, 1950.

165. Shinners, B. M., and Hamby, W. B. "The results of surgical removal of protruded lumbar intervertebral discs." *J. Neurosurg.*, 1:117, 1944.

166. ———. "Protruded lumbar intervertebral discs: results following surgical and nonsurgical therapy." *J. Neurosurg.*, 6:450, 1949.

167. Simpson, W. J., and Orange, R. P. "Total body scanning with strontium–85 in the diagnosis of metastatic bone disease." *Canad. Med. Assn. J.*, 93:1237, 1965.

168. Sissons, H. A. "Tumors of the Vertebral Column," in *Modern Trends in Diseases of the Vertebral Column*, Butterworth and Co. Ltd., 1959, 192–209.

169. Slepian, A. "Lumbar-disc surgery: long-term follow-up results from three neurosurgeons." *New York J. Med.*, 66:1063–68, May, 1966.

170. Spurling, R. G. *Lesions of the lumbar intervertebral disc*, 2nd ed. I, 1–30, Charles Thomas, 1953.

171. ———. "Diagnosis of disc lesions." *American Academy of Orthopaedic Surgeons Instructional Course Lectures*, vol. 1, Ann Arbor: J. W. Edwards, 1943, 109.

172. Spurling, R. G., and Grantham, D. "The end results of surgery for ruptured intervertebral discs." *J. Neurosurg.*, 6:57, 1949.

173. Spurling, R. G., and Scoville, W. B. "Lateral rupture of the cervical intervertebral discs: a common cause of shoulder and arm pain." *Surg. Gyne. & Obst.* 78:350, 1944.

174. Spurling, R. G., and Segerberg, L. H. "Lateral intervertebral disc lesions in the lower cervical region." *JAMA*, 151:354, 1953.

175. Steindler, A. *Diseases and deformities of the spine and thorax*. St. Louis: C. V. Mosby Co., 1929.

176. Steindler, A. "Differential diagnosis of pain low in the back." *JAMA*, 110:106, 1938.

177. ———. "The interpretation of the pain syndromes in lumbosacralgia." *American Academy of Orthopaedic Surgeons Instructional Course Lectures*, vol. XIV, Ann Arbor: J. W. Edwards, 1957, 11.

178. ———. "The pathomechanics of the sacrolumbar junction." *American Academy of Orthopaedic Surgeons Instructional Course Lectures*, vol. XII, Ann Arbor: J. W. Edwards, 1955, 117.

179. Stinchfield, F. E., and Gruess, R. L. "Indications for spine fusion in conjunction with removal of herniated nucleus pulposus." *American Academy of Orthopaedic Surgeons Instructional Course Lectures*, vol. XVIII, St. Louis: C.V. Mosby Co., 1961, 41.

180. Sylven B. "On the biology of nucleus pulposus." *Acta Ortho. Scandinavia*, 20:275–79, 1950.

181. Teng, P., and Papatheodorou, C. "Lumbar spondylosis with compression of cauda equina." *Arch. Neurol.*, 8:221–29, February, 1963.

182. Thiobodeau, A. A. "Closed space infection following removal of lumbar intervertebral disc." *Clin. Neurosurg.*, (William & Wilkins, Baltimore) 14:337–60, 1967.

183. Trowbridge, W. V., and French, J. D. "False positive lumbar myelography." *Neurology*, 4:339–44, 1954.

184. Thompson, F. R. "Examination of the back." *American Academy of Orthopaedic Surgeons Instructional Course Lectures*, vol. IX, Ann Arbor: J. W. Edwards, 1952, 31.

185. Valls, J., Otolenghi, C. E., and Schajowicz, F. "Aspiration biopsy in diagnosis of lesions of vertebral bodies." *JAMA*, 136:376, 1948.

186. Verbiest, H. "A radicular syndrome from developmental narrowing of the lumbar vertebral canal." *J. Bone Jt. Surg.*, 36B:230–37, May, 1954.

187. Walker, H. R. "Extradural osseous lesions simulating the disc syndrome." *JAMA*, 172:691–94, Feb., 1960.

188. Waris, W. "Lumbar-disc herniations: clinical studies and late results." *Acta Chir. Scandinavia*, Supplement 140, 1948.

189. Watkins, A. L. "Electromyography in orthopedics." *J. Bone Jt Surg.*, 31A:822–29, No. 4, October, 1949.

190. Wetzel, N., Arieff, A., and Tungbay, E. "Retroperitoneal lumbar and pelvic malignancies simulating the disc syndrome." *Arch. of Surg.*, 86:1069–71, June, 1963.

191. Welkin, J. S., and Hoke, G. G. "Comparative studies of discography and myelography." *Radiology*, 64:704–712, 1955.

192. Whiteleather, J. E., Semmes, R. E., and Murphey, F. "The roentgenographic signs of herniation of the cervical intervertebral disc." *Radiology*, 46:213, 1946.

193. Wiberg, G. "Back pain in relation to the nerve supply of the intervertebral disc." *Acta Ortho. Scandinavia*, 19:211–221, 1949.

194. Williams, P. C. "The diagnosis and conservative management of lesions of the lumbosacral spine." *American Academy of Orthopaedic Surgeons Instructional Course Lectures*, vol. IV, Ann Arbor: J. W. Edwards, 1947.

195. ———. "The conservative management of lesions of the lumbosacral spine." *American Academy of Orthopaedic Surgeons Instructional Course Lectures*, vol. X, Ann Arbor: J. W. Edwards, 1952, 90.

196. ———. "Reduced lumbosacral joint space: its relation to sciatic irritation." *JAMA*, 99:1677, 1932.

197. ———. "Lesions of the lumbosacral spine: acute traumatic destruction of lumbosacral intervertebral disc." *J. Bone Jt. Surg.*, 19:343, 1937.

198. Williams, P. C., and Yglesias, L. "Lumbosacral facetectomy for post-fusion persistent sciatics." *J. Bone Jt. Surg.*, 15:579–590, 1933.

199. Willis, T. A. "An analysis of vertebral anomalies." *Am. J. Surg.*, 6:163, 1929.

200. ———. "Low-back pain: the anatomical structure of the lumbar region, including variations." *J. Bone Jt. Surg.*, 19:745, 1937.

201. ———. "Abnormal anatomy of the lumbosacral region with reference to low back pain." *American Academy of Orthopaedic Surgeons Instructional Course Lectures*, vol. V, Ann Arbor: J. W. Edwards, 1948, 276.

202. Wilson, J. C., Jr. "Degenerative arthritis of the lumbosacral joint: the end-space lesion." *JAMA*, 169:1437–42, March, 1959.

203. ———. "Degenerative arthritis of lumbar intervertebral joints: a clinical study." *Am. J. Surg.*, 100:313–22, August 1960.

204. Young, H. H., and Love, J. G. "End results of removal of protruded lumbar intervertebral discs with and without fusion." *American Academy of Orthopaedic Surgeons Instructional Course Lectures*, vol. XVI, Ann Arbor: J. W. Edwards, 1959, 213.

205. Young, H. H., Love, J. G., Svien, H. J., Price, R. D., and Kroll, H. G. "Low-back and sciatic pain: long-term results after removal of protruded intervertebral disc with and without fusion." *Clin. Ortho.*, vol. 5, 128–37, 1959.

206. Young, J. H. "Cervical and thoracic intervertebral disc disease." *M. J. Australia*, 2:833, 1946.

207. Young, R. H. "Protrusion of the intervertebral discs." *Proc. Roy. Soc. Med.*, 40:233:236, 1947.

208. Young, J. M., and Funk, F. J. "Incidence of tumor metastasis to the lumbar spine: a comparative study of roentgenographic changes and gross lesions." *J. Bone Jt. Surg.* 35A:55–64, Jan., 1953.

209. Silver, Richard A. "Intermittent claudication of neuro-spinal origin." *Arch. Surg.*, vol. 98, April, 1969, 523–529.

210. Silver, Richard A., and Krempen, John F. "Removal of iliac bone for bone grafting in back fusions." *Ortho. Review*, vol. VIII, 2, February, 1979.

211. ———. "An analysis of differential epidural spinal anesthesia and pentothal: pain study in differential diagnosis of back pain." *Spine*, vol. 4, 5, Sept/Oct., 1979.

212. ———. "Ligamentum flavotomy." *Ortho Review*, vol. VIII, 9, Sept., 1979.

213. ———. "Pedicle fat grafts in lumbar spine surgery: evaluation of a method to prevent cicatrix formation." Paper presented at the American Academy of Orthopaedic Surgeons Convention, Las Vegas, Nevada, Feb., 1981.

214. ———. "Selective lumbar and cervical nerve root injection studies, methods

for evaluating radicular symptoms.'' *J. Neuro. & Ortho. Surg.*, vol. 2, issue 3, October, 1981.

215. Silver, Richard A., Krempen, John F., Clymer, O., and Kaubisch, D. ''Left common iliac arterial aneurysm causing L5 nerve root symptoms secondary to injury following laminectomy.'' *J. Neuro. & Ortho. Surg.*, vol. 3, issue 3, October, 1982.

7. The Use of Videotechnology by the Medical Trial Defense Bar—A Case Study

James B. Couch, M.D., J.D., F.C.L.M.

I. INTRODUCTION—THE VIDEO GENERATION

The large segment of humanity in this country born between the end of World War II and the beginning of the Vietnam War, often referred to as the "baby boomers," may more descriptively be characterized as "the video generation." The youngest members of this group are just entering the work force, while its more senior representatives have begun to acquire some political and economic power. This will truly be a segment of society to reckon with in the next twenty to thirty years.

To a significant extent, what this group has in common, even across socio-economic, cultural, ethnic, and political lines, is that it represents the first generation to be born and bred on video. From "Romper Room" to "The Muppet Show," from Milton Berle to David Letterman, from Chip'n Dale to the Chippendales, this generation has been profoundly influenced by the visual medium.

This group, more than any other before it, has come to depend on video for a major part of its collective education. Modern videotechnology has brought to the small screen everything from quarks to quasers. With state-of-the-art graphics, photographic techniques, and expert commentary, this generation has come to recognize how powerful an educator this "professor of the air waves" can be.

Video can provide interesting and often unique methods of illustrating facts about our world of which we might otherwise remain ignorant. It can clarify some of the hidden truths of existence, if used judiciously. On the other hand, it can also trick or deceive us by distorting reality in ways of which we are unaware.

So video, like so many other tools of modern technology, has the potential to be either an inimitable educator or an habitual obfuscator. Its potential value as a clarifier or facilitator in the truth-finding process in modern-day litigation must be measured in that light.

II. GENERAL RATIONALE FOR THE USE OF VIDEOTECHNOLOGY IN THE COURTROOM

In today's world of increasingly complex, technologically oriented, civil trial truth-finding, it would almost seem to be a given that videotechnology could and perhaps even should play a vital role. For one thing, civil litigation is becoming almost prohibitively expensive in highly technical areas like medical malpractice and products liability. Any tool that could be judiciously used to clarify facts or processes that might otherwise require even more time-consuming and costly alternatives should be welcome.

But what of the impact on a jury of something other than the "genuine article" (assuming that it exists), i.e., a video substitute? Will efforts to insure accuracy and authenticity minimize the dramatic impact of the visual medium and dilute the emotional impression intended for jurors' minds?

In a major study supported by the National Science Foundation, investigators from the Department of Communication at Michigan State University evaluated the effects of videotaped testimony or information processing and decision making in jury trials. They concluded that . . . "there is no evidence to suggest that the uses of videotape exerts any deleterious effects on the juror responses studied; in fact, as far as retention of trial-related information is concerned, it appears that videotaped testimony sometimes results in higher retention levels." [Miller, G.R., and F.S. Siebert, *Effects of Videotaped Testimony on Information Processing and Decision-making in Jury Trials: Final Report*; NSF Grant #GI 38398 (December, 1975)] The fact that the study is ten years old, rather than detracting from its credibility, only enhances it, for at least two reasons:

1. Videotechnology now has the capacity to be much more realistic and interesting; and
2. Today's juror is more accustomed to this type of medium.

Since this technology is worthy of serious consideration for inclusion in select trials, in this chapter the general uses to which it may be put in the courtroom shall be examined. In addition, there will be an analysis of the specific ways in which trial lawyers may use this tool on behalf of their clients, as well as a detailed discussion of how it has been successfully applied by the author in a multimillion-dollar case. The chapter will conclude with some practical considerations, and recommendations for further development of this important new technology in the courtroom setting.

III. TWO GENERAL EVIDENTIARY USES OF VIDEOTECHNOLOGY AT TRIAL

A. *To Show Relevance*

1. *Definitional Purpose*

As an initial proposition, evidence must be relevant to be admissible. For a videotaped rendition of a person, event, process, or environment to be relevant, such a product must serve to prove a material issue or issues in dispute in a case in an accurate, authentic, and cost-effective manner.

2. *Medical Litigation Examples*

The classical way that plaintiffs' attorneys in medical malpractice cases have satisfied the relevancy hurdle in the past has been to produce so-called ''Day in the Life'' videotapes of injured plaintiffs (particularly infants and small children). These videotapes are relevant inasmuch as they demonstrate the extent of damages, from both a cosmetic and functional standpoint, to the plaintiffs owing to the alleged negligence of the defendants.

Medical defense attorneys have been reluctant to use this technology, even as a counterweight to the potentially dramatic impact of a videotape of this sort produced by the plaintiff. However, just as surely as a plaintiff may use a ''Day in the Life'' video to ''prove'' damages, so too could a defense attorney use a videotape of the environment in which the alleged negligence occurred to illustrate, among other things, the applicable standard of care, also a material issue for proof in a personal injury action.

This ''creation of an environment'' use for a videotape on behalf of medical malpractice defendants will be discussed in significant detail in the case-study analysis below. Suffice it to say that in that case applying this technology proved to be much less costly, disruptive, and time-consuming in achieving its evidentiary purpose than the alternative—a jury viewing of ''the scene'' (i.e., a university hospital neonatal intensive care unit).

B. *To Assess Credibility*

1. *Definitional Purpose*

The other major function that videotape technology may have in the courtroom is that of permitting an assessment of credibility (i.e., the believability of an event, test, process, or causal connection) that otherwise might not be demonstrable in an equally effective manner.

2. *Videotape-facilitated Credibility Assessment*

As far as testing is concerned, there are at least six criteria upon which credibility may be assessed:

a) Personal knowledge;
b) Recollection;
c) Perception;

d) Intention;
e) State of mind; and
f) Operation of mind.

Videotaped testimony may facilitate an assessment of how well a witness, defendant, or expert measures up to all of these criteria. Moreover, the judicious use of a zoom lens may even permit a more accurate assessment of credibility concerning such criteria as state of mind than could ever be achieved in its absence. Clearly, this might have significant implications in such important matters as contract execution, testamentary recitals, and witness depositions in civil and criminal proceedings.

IV. SPECIFIC EVIDENTIARY OBJECTIONS TO THE USE OF VIDEOTECHNOLOGY AT TRIAL

A. *Lack of Relevance*

1. *Objection*

A videotape could be objected to as not being admissible as a means of proving or clarifying one or more of the issues in a case.

2. *Response*

In most situations, especially under the Federal Rules of Evidence that are increasingly being adopted by state courts, this objection could be answered if the attorney could demonstrate that a videotape could be helpful in proving a material issue in cases such as:

a) *Causation*: In *Szeliga v. General Motors Corp.*, 723 F.2d 566 (1st Cir. 1984), the circuit court held that the trial judge did not err in finding films prepared by the manufacturer and offered to support its theory that a wheel fell off because of impact (and not because of the loss of lug nuts) to be more probative than prejudicial.
b) *Damages*: In *Conti v. Ford Motor Co.*, 578 F.Supp. 1429 (E.D. Pa. 1983), the court confirmed a jury's award of damages when a car manufactured by the defendant unexpectedly moved forward; and
c) *Standard of Care/Contributory Negligence*: In *Abernathy v. Superior Hardwoods, Inc.*, 704 F.2d, 963 (7th Cir. 1983), the court found no error in a videotape depicting how logs were to be loaded in support of a contributory negligence claim.

B. *Biased, Prejudicial and Inflammatory Evidence*

1. *Objection*

Even if a videotape is relevant on any of the foregoing bases, its potential for creating a biased, prejudicial, or inflammatory impression on the jury may outweigh its probabtive value.

2. *Response*

This involves a balancing of the probative versus the prejudicial nature of the videotaped evidence and is a matter for determination to be left to the sound discretion of the trial judge. In all of the cases discussed in the previous section, the trial court was upheld in making the determination that the probative value of the videotapes outweighed any prejudicial effect.

C. *Not the Best Evidence*

1. *Objections*

The objection here would be that having the witness in courts or permitting a jury viewing of a scene would be the "best evidence."

2. *Response*

This may be answered in Pennsylvania as well as in many other states simply by reference to a civil rule or rules. Pa. R. Civ. P. 4017.1, effective April 1, 1973, provides for videotape depositions of a medical witness or any witness called as an expert other than a party at trial for any purpose.

D. *Lack of Authenticity*

1. *Objection*

This objection states that a particular videotape is not a "fair" and "truthful" representation of the object, person, or place in question.

2. *Response*

It is not necessary to call upon a photographer to testify as to a videotape's accuracy. However, in light of the possibility that a videotape might be misleadingly edited, it may be prudent to have the cameraman under subpoena, or at least someone such as the producer, director, scriptwriter or other such witness under oath to testify as to the authenticity of a videotape as being a fair and truthful representation of reality.

E. *Hearsay*

1. *Objection*

Any audio portion, titles, captions, graphs, charts, and tables may be construed as out-of-court statements offered to prove the truth of a material fact in issue. An alternative objection is that these verbal messages may be more appropriately the subject of expert testimony.

2. *Response*

Verbal messages in a videotape need not be fatal to its admissibility as objectionable hearsay. If all the verbal messages on a videotape representing statements, treatises, expert testimony, and the like have already been admitted into evidence without objection, then any such verbal message should not be excluded as hearsay. Still, it might be a good idea to play back the video without sound and have an expert witness (or a witness familiar with the subject of the videotape or actively involved in its production) serve as a narrator. Any need for captions, titles, charts, and graphs may also be minimized in this way.

F. *Cumulative Evidence*

1. *Objection*

As a follow-up to the above response, an objection may be raised that if all a videotape accomplishes is to reiterate material already in evidence, while avoiding a hearsay objection, it could be excluded as cumulative.

2. *Response*

It is not impossible to escape this potential double bind, but it takes some creativity on the part of the producer of the videotape (who should be present at the time of the videotape's introduction into evidence).

The facts, testimony, or processes in question, as well as the material covered on the videotape may already be in evidence when it is sought to be shown. Nevertheless, one of the major functions of the videotape is to permit the graphic illustration of facts, settings, or processes in a way otherwise not practicable. Thus, although the message sought to be conveyed by the videotape may not amount to anything not already in evidence, the method of presenting the message may be different and hopefully more effective, and thus, not objectionable as cumulative evidence.

V. CONCEIVING OF THE SPECIFIC ROLE OF A VIDEOTAPE IN YOUR CASE

A. *Deciding Whether to Use a Videotape*

This often depends upon the type of case. Although videotechnology is flexible enough to be used in many areas of litigation, insofar as its ability to make a unique contribution to a trial is concerned it only lends itself to a select few.

There are always alternatives to videotapes, including (but not limited to): photographs, slides, acetate overlays, overhead projections or films. From a cost standpoint, perhaps each of these alternatives would cost less and be less time-consuming than a videotape.

Accordingly, videotapes must be reserved for only those few cases in which the time- and cost-investment involved are deemed "worth it" to all concerned. In other words, it should be considered that the purpose(s) sought to be accomplished will be best served through the impact of videotechnology on the judge and jury.

B. *Purposes for Which a Videotape Would be Appropriate*

There are many uses for videotape during a trial. Among them are:

1. To prove an important part of a case in the most effective way, including (but not limited to):
   a) Facts (e.g., spatial relationships not otherwise proveable except through disputed testimony);
   b) The standard of care or contributory negligence (through the re-creation of the environment at issue in a sufficiently realistic way not otherwise obtainable by alternative audiovisual methods);
   c) Legal and proximate causation (through computerized reconstruction of accidents, etc.); and
   d) Damages (through "Day in the Life" videos).
2. To refute opposing witness' testimony with demonstrative evidence;

3. To supplement or corroborate illustratively a key witness' testimony;
4. As a jury psychological counterweight to the other side's videotape;
5. To rekindle judge and juror interest at a critical time in a trial (e.g., before closing arguments); and
6. As part of a summation.

Clearly, a videotape should satisfy at least one of the first four purposes listed under #1 above. In most situations, depending on the amount of cost and time involved, to justify its use for trial it should probably satisfy at least one or more of reasons 2 through 6, also.

VI. THE MAKING OF A MEDICAL DEFENSE VIDEOTAPE—A CASE STUDY

Assuming that the decision has been made, based on the foregoing, to "take the video plunge," how does one go about accomplishing it in terms of one's own case? The following section will demonstrate this step-by-step through a case study of a videotape produced by the author that recreated the environment of a university hospital neonatal intensive care unit out of which a multimillion-dollar, brain-damaged baby case was brought. This videotape was used successfully in the case, which resulted in a jury verdict for all defendants (the hospital, two neonatologists, and one pediatric resident). [Cf. L.A.M.P. 13(1):5–7 (1/85)].

A. *Background of the Case*

At 3:46 A.M. on June 14, 1978, the mother in this case gave birth vaginally to a breech-presenting, 2 lb., 9 oz., twelve-week-premature baby girl following five-and-one-half days of prematurely ruptured membranes. The mother had had a history of intermittent bleeding in the first and second trimesters, and had had a history of exposure to DES in utero, for which she had been treated by a specialist in DES-associated reproductive anomalies for several years. She had had one previous miscarriage and, prior to that, a seven-year history of inability to conceive.

The infant was pale, floppy, and not breathing following traumatic vaginal birth performed by an OB-GYN resident (instead of a cesarean section done by the attending physician, since an ultrasound the previous day had revealed a "probably nonviable infant weighing about a pound.")

The infant's one-minute Apgar score was 1. Vigorous resuscitation improved her Apgar score to 6 by five minutes. Despite this, the infant had to be intubated at around 4:00 A.M., following transfer from the delivery suite to the adjacent neonatal intensive care unit at the university hospital. There she was attended by a third-year pediatric resident on-call (as she had been from the moment of birth), as well as various neonatal intensive-care unit (NICU) nurses.

Due to continuing poor blood gases despite 40 percent F_1O_2 and PEEP, the oxygen concentration was raised to 70 percent. Early that morning, the infant's pO_2 was elevated to 190 mm Hg (or about twice that recommended by a 1977 manual of the American Academy of Pediatrics.) Her blood levels were brought back to the recommended range within about five hours.

The child suffered a stormy two-month course in the intensive care nursery, but she was able to be discharged at two months of age. However, at the time of discharge, she was beginning to exhibit problems with visual fixation compatible with incipient retrolental fibrophasia (RLF), which eventually blinded her. Subsequently, she experienced severe developmental retardation. Ultimately, in January of 1980, she was diagnosed by a pediatric neurodevelopmentalist as suffering from severe cerebral palsy.

The plaintiff's attorney brought an action alleging at least $5 million in compensable damages, allegedly having resulted from the negligence of two neonatologists, the pediatric resident, and others working in the NICU. The case was tried to a jury of seven women and five men in a five-week trial. The trial included the admission into evidence of both the plaintiff's "Day in the Life" and the defendants "NICU Environment Recreation" videotapes. As late as three hours prior to the jury verdict, the plaintiffs refused an offer of $2.2 million (advanced by a representative of the state's Catastrophic Loss Fund) to settle. The jury then returned a verdict of "no liability" on the part of any of the four defendants.

B. *Medical Defense Strategy*

The foregoing case was meticulously prepared by defense counsel over a three-and-one-half-year period. The work included extensive searches through medical literature, pleadings, depositions, and ordinary and expert witness preparation. However, the defense still lacked the ability to effectively communicate in the courtroom the nature of the medical environment in which the alleged negligence occurred. The author first suggested the videotaping of the NICU during the first year of the litigation, while he was working as a resident physician in a medical intensive care unit.

Other types of visual demonstrative evidence were considered along the way, such as photographs, slides, or movies. It was decided to go with the more expensive videotape alternative in this important case for the following reasons:

1. A "moving picture" (as opposed to photographs or slides) was necessary to demonstrate the fast pace of the NICU and procedures being performed;
2. A videotape, rather than a film, conveyed more of the sense of realism to which jurors were accustomed through television news reporting; and
3. The plaintiff had produced a videotape.

The following section will describe in significant detail how to produce a videotape like that of the author in this case. Ways in which the attorney trying the case, as well as medical defendants, witnesses, and experts, may participate in the production process will be discussed in this context.

C. *The Production of the Videotape*

1. *The Preproduction Stage*

a) *The Script—The Blueprint*

The script is the blueprint from which the videotape is produced. It should be written by someone well acquainted with the environment in which the videotape will be shot.

The scriptwriter first must rough out an outline of the script presenting the general content of what the videotape is intended to convey. The general parameters of the videotape must be established during this initial drafting. The videotape should be limited to 10 to 15 minutes in length. Anything longer than this will be longer than the optimal attention span of the viewer.

The videotape script should, if possible, be written so that it is comprehensible to the least well-educated juror. If done properly, it may serve as the sole source of a clear understanding on the jury's part of the relevant environment in a case arising out of a complex setting. At this stage, it might be advisable to consult with software specialists in the production of videotapes in medical and other technical areas. The author did this for this case, working closely with them to produce a videotape of the university hospital's NICU that was both accurate and understandable.

b) *The Video Storyboard*

After the initial script has been roughed out, the next step is to produce the so-called video storyboard. Video storyboarding permits the synchronization of the script narrative with the accompanying visual displays.

Even if the videotape is not ultimately played with an accompanying narrative, video storyboarding is an integral part of the preproduction process. Video storyboarding determines the sequence, duration, and pacing of each visual display, comprising the videotape as a whole. How each of these elements is to be organized must be established prior to the shooting. Video storyboarding permits the matching of visual display to the accompanying narrated script (whether or not there is background narration presented at trial as opposed to live narration by witnesses).

It is this part of the preproduction process that requires the closest coordination between the attorney, medical client, and professional videotape corporation (producer, director, scriptwriters, etc.); this is the heart and soul of the videotape to be presented to judge and jurors. Moreover, if background narration is omitted (to avoid hearsay on other evidentiary objections), then the medical client may well serve as the "live narrator" of the videotape (as occurred in this case). Although the defendant should not be permitted to govern how the videotape is produced, he or she should at least be made aware of the general content, sequencing, and pacing of the videotape at this juncture, especially if his or her "live narration" at trial is to be reasonably anticipated.

c) *Staging and Casting*

Whenever an on-site shooting is to occur in a hospital setting, the prerequisite administrative clearances and approvals must be obtained. To acquire even as little as ten-to-fifteen minutes of useful videotape usually take up to a full day's work on site.

At a minimum, to bring an out-of-house production crew with cameras, lighting, meters and cables into a setting as rife with potential liability as NICU, the following should be obtained:

i) Administration approval from the hospital's chief executive officer or his designate;
ii) Legal approval from the hospital's in-house or out-of-house counsel;
iii) Medical approval from the director of the NICU;
iv) Proof of liability insurance coverage from the production company;
v) Assurance that the confidentiality of all medical records, physician-patient transactions, or medical incidents observed will be maintained;
vi) Informed consent to the shooting of any infants from the neck up; and
vii) Model releases to be distributed and signed by all persons appearing on the videotape to protect the videographer, his agents, and principals in case of any distribution of the product that might result in "ridicule, reproach, scorn or indignity."

d) *Sound Preparation*

If there is to be narration, then this should be prepared prior to the shoot, preferably in a professional sound studio. The narrator should be someone already under subpoena so that he or she may be cross-examined at trial for any statements made on the videotape. Ideally, the person should be familiar with the case and be competent (i.e., an expert) to testify independently on the matters discussed in the narrative. In this particular case, a nurse already under subpoena who had been involved in the care of the infant was the narrator. For a discussion of how the finished videotape was then presented at trial, please refer to subpart D, below.

A day or so prior to the actual shooting, the production crew, accompanied by either the attorney, medical client, or both, should visit the shooting facility to establish the setting and staging formats. The precise areas to be shot should be scouted to determine in advance the precise logistics involved in shooting the visuals of the videotape. The cast of characters to appear (with or without speaking or active parts) should be selected, if at all possible, during this "reconnaissance mission,'' prior to the day of the shoot. They should be made aware of their parts, and how they will ''fit into'' the videotape as a whole.

e) *Quality Assurance*

Judge and jurors alike are accustomed to the level of video quality they see on the evening news on television. Anything less than this will probably fail to communicate effectively enough.

For this reason, at least for cases such the one under discussion, with potentially large liability exposure, it is more cost-effective to obtain broadcast quality videotape. This is usually only obtainable by use of three-tube, professional video cameras; 3/4-inch master videotapes; proper lighting, and other accessories; and the use of professional production crews with experience in the shooting of medical settings.

2. *The Production Stage—The Day of the Shoot*

a) *The Coordination of the Cast*

All persons (professional and amateur) to appear in the videotape should be accounted for at the outset, and some reasonable idea given them as to when and how long they will be expected to appear. Model releases should be signed at this time.

b) *Logistical/Safety Considerations*

The movements of the cast of characters and the production crew, with all its cameras, lighting, and cables, should be coordinated by a director intimately familar with the videotape production process in general, as well as the particular sequences and pacing of the videotape to be shot. The movements of these parties must be coordinated so as to accomplish the production of the videotape without undue interference with the normal operation of the neonatal intensive care unit.

c) *Authenticity Considerations*

It is impossible to recreate the environment exactly as it might have been at the time of the incident that is the subject of the suit. For example, in this case the shooting occurred years after the actual incident took place and during the day shift (as opposed to the wee hours of the morning, when the infant in question was delivered). Nevertheless, the authenticity of the videotape is an important factor in both its admissibility and impact, and must be sought to the extent possible.

When recreating an environment as sophisticated as a neonatal intensive care unit, certain aspects of it are bound to have changed during the time between the incident and the shooting itself. To preserve authenticity, as great an effort as possible should be made only to shoot those technologies in existence at the time of the incident. If this proves to be impossible or very impractical, then whoever narrates the videotape script should account for these differences when explaining the visual displays.

Of course, the pacing, sequencing, and actual events videotaped will also vary from what actually occurred. To the extent it may be required (i.e., in response to an objection by the other side at trial), these differences should also be explained. The important point is that the videotape produced give the judge and jury a birds-eye view of what occurs in a neonatal intensive care unit on a typical day, if not necessarily the precise day the incident occurred.

This important distinction should be made at the outset, since it goes to the heart of the purpose for admitting the videotape into evidence; that is, to give the judge and jury an audiovisual education on how things occur, and the ways in which health care personnel must respond to these occurrences, in a modern university hospital NICU such as the one in which the allegedly negligent act or acts took place. This audiovisual education, if it achieves its purpose, should help elucidate, in a way that expert testimony never could, the standard of care provided sick, severely premature infants in such a setting.

If the preproduction format has been followed religiously, the actual shooting of the videotape should proceed smoothly, excepting unforeseen circumstances. On the set, each participant should have a discrete and well-understood set of functions to fulfill to make the shooting most effective.

The scriptwriter (and, to the extent possible, the attorney and/or medical client) should always be present to insure that what is being shot by the videographer (or cameraman) makes sense in the context of the accompanying narrative (i.e., that the video storyboard is followed to the letter). The director or producer should communicate the information provided by the scriptwriter, attorney, and medical client directly to the cameraman. The director will also be in charge of coordinating the cameraman and other technicians with the actors or other participants in the videotape itself.

If the foregoing format is followed and the overall coordination of the videotape is well accomplished, the final product should achieve the intended medical, legal, and evidentiary results in a logical, comprehensible, interesting, and authentic way that is neither biased, prejudicial, or inflammatory. The intended purpose of the presentation may be spelled out or narrated "live" at the beginning and reiterated at the end of the videotape, to the extent that doing so is not objectionable as hearsay or cumulative evidence.

3. *The Postproduction or Editing Stage*

Once the shooting and narration (if any) are completed, the important process of editing begins. Postproduction involves editing, crediting, and titling, to complete the videotape production package. Editing should be done in a professional studio. At the very least, the attorney, scriptwriter, cameramen, and, if possible, the coordinating producer should be present during this important process.

Initially, all of the footage should be shot and timed. The footage should then be roughly coordinated with the audio portion (whether this involves narration, background music, or whatever). The editing process begins in earnest then, when the visual footage is electronically "cut and spliced" to synchronize precisely with the script envisioned by the scriptwriter, attorney, and medical client at the video storyboarding preproduction stage. Following this, the appropriate titling, character generation, computer graphics, or animation maybe inserted at the preconceived times in the videotape. Credits concerning the writers, producers, directors, and facilities used may be added at the end, but are generally omitted until after the videotape has fulfilled its evidentiary purposes at trial.

Editing to produce the final videotape package, however, is much more than a matter of "cutting and splicing." It is at the heart of the postproduction process, out of which emerges the final product. It is for that reason that the attorney, as well as the scriptwriter and cameramen are indispensable participants in this process.

The editing process should be onto a 3/4-inch master videotape. Fluidity of presentation is of great importance since judge and jurors are accustomed to and expect "broadcast quality" videotape productions. Editors of the videotape should put themselves in the judge and jurors' shoes to insure that the final product is both accurate and understandable in the communication of its intended messages.

Overall timing and pacing is important in this respect. However, authenticity of presentation must never be compromised in making the videotape "more interesting" to its intended viewers. Otherwise, the entire videotape may be rejected as evidence. Also, titles, clients, graphs, and narration must be used very carefully to avoid objections of hearsay, or that the evidence is cumulative or usurps the expert witness' function. Hearsay objections may be answered by having the declarants of any statements (such as those made by a narrator) under subpoena and cross-examinable. Any titling, graphs, or charts would not usurp the expert witness' function so long as the messages conveyed are already admitted into evidence through an expert. Finally, any graphics, charts, or titles would not be cumulative evidence, since they would be admissible to clarify in a unique way information that had already been admitted through an expert.

Once the videotape package has been fully edited, all relevant parties (attorneys, medical client, experts, scriptwriter, producer/director, and camaramen/editor) should review the final product. After this, any last-minute changes that might help to insure accuracy, authenticity, and efficiency in communicating the intended messages and achieve the desired purposes should be made. Copies of the final 3/4-inch master videotape may then be copied onto either 1/2-inch VHS or Beta Max formats, depending upon which is compatible with the VCR to be used at the time of trial.

VII. USE OF THE VIDEOTAPE AT TRIAL

A. *Strategic/Tactical Considerations—Whether To Use It or Not*

The availability of a broadcast quality videotape still doesn't compel its use at trial. The most experienced trial lawyers know that the best-laid plans may have to be jettisoned on very short notice, depending upon the conduct of the trial. In complicated trials such as the one in question, strategies and tactics may have to be altered (often significantly) from moment to moment, not to mention from day to day.

B. *Timing is Crucial*

The timing of the videotape presentation at trial is of critical importance as far as the psychology of judge and jury persuasion is concerned. As discussed previously, to avoid hearsay, cumulative evidence, and competency objections, the videotape probably should be admitted after the defense experts have testified.

In our case, it was used near the end of our direct examination of our client, the NICU director. Since our client was director of the NICU at both the time of the incident and the videotape shooting, she was, with the videotape audio turned down able to comment upon changes that had occurred in the NICU between the two times, thus insuring the video's authenticity. As a witness available for cross-examination (and an expert witness, as well), our neonatologist client was competent to comment upon the visual and verbal messages conveyed by the videotape. Since all these verbal and visual messages (including graphics) had already been put into evidence without objection either through our experts or in the form of admissible medical literature, our client was free to explain how the visual aides clarified key medicolegal issues discussed previously (and esoterically) by medical experts.

Finally, and perhaps most importantly, our NICU director client was able to corroborate under oath the authenticity of the videotapes as to the relative size of the infants, the procedures performed on the infants, and the level of care and compassion involved in typical NICU care. It was perhaps the vivid demonstration of this human touch existing amid the maze of sophisticated medical technology comprising a modern NICU that helped convey most to the judge and jury the dedication and integrity of those involved in the care of severely premature infants, far better than any experts ever could have by themselves.

VIII. SOME FINAL CONSIDERATIONS

A. *Time Involved in Production*

As the foregoing discussion concerning the production of a customized videotape for use at trial on behalf of medical clients has no doubt conveyed, the use of videotapes as a form of demonstrative evidence is not for the faint of heart. It involves a very significant commitment of time and energy for all concerned. In this particular case, it took about 200 man-hours to put together what was ultimately only a ten-minute-long presentation at trial. Considering that the attorney representing the medical client should be involved in perhaps 1/3 to 1/2 of these total man-hours, it is clear that the costs of just his or her time, not to mention that of all the other parties involved in the production, will be quite substantial.

A rule of thumb in the industry is that the overall cost of customized broadcast quality videotapes in highly sophisticated areas such as medical technology starts at about $1,000 per minute. Depending upon the amount of computer graphics, animation, and other extras, the rate may be as much as two to three times this much.

B. *A Matter of Propriety*

Based on these foregoing time and cost estimates, it is clear that the client and his or her insurance carrier should be intimately involved in deciding whether to undertake what would be a major project in any trial. The message here is: *Be Selective*! There are actually very few cases in a medical malpractice defense firm's office that even lend themselves to videotape production for trial, much less justify the amount of time and cost involved.

Nevertheless, there are certain very significant cases, such as the one discussed in this chapter, which may satisfy the imposing requirements of propriety of purpose and magnitude of potential liability exposure to justify the undertaking of a medical defense videotape for trial. Done correctly, it can be an invaluable educational tool in the successful defense of medical clients in very significant and complicated cases. Undertaken in less appropriate cases, it can not only be a monumental waste of time and money, but, even more devastatingly, it can become a definite hindrance to the overall successful defense strategy.

IX. CONCLUSIONS

A. *Summary*

1. *General Evidentiary Uses of Videotapes*

Videotapes may be used in the courtroom for two general evidentiary purposes: to help prove material issues in the most effective way, and to determine credibility.

2. *Objections*

There may be several objections to the use of videotapes for these purposes, viz:

a) Its lack of relevance;
b) Its not being the "best evidence";
c) Its lack of authenticity;
d) Its being hearsay (especially if accompanied by verbal messages);

e) Its bias, prejudice, or inflammatory nature; and/or
f) Its cumulative nature.

3. *A Case Study*

   In this chapter, a case study was presented in detail, with a view to how a defense videotape could be produced in a trial similar to that in which the author was involved. The background of the case, the theories of liability, the defense strategies, and the role and production of a customized videotape were covered. The role of the defense attorney and his or her medical client in the production of the videotape was discussed at each step of the process.

4. *Strategies for Use at Trial*

   Strategic and tactical considerations concerning whether to use the videotape, once produced, at trial, and, if so, when to present to greatest advantage for a medical client, were all discussed. How to minimize objection and maximize impact when using this technology was analyzed in some depth.

5. *Practical Considerations*

   Finally, some time and cost considerations from both the attorney's and medical client's perspective were discussed. The thrust of the discussion was that videotape production such as that successfully applied in this case involved in the neighborhood of 200 man-hours and costs in the $1,000 per minute range. Attorneys and their medical clients should be very selective in deciding whether the merits and potential liability exposure of their cases can justify this amount of time and expense.

B. *Recommendations*

1. *Know the Uses and Limitations of (and Potential Objections to) Videotape in the Courtroom*: Every step of the videotaping process, from initial conceptualization to implementation at trial, must be governed by these considerations.
2. *Know What is Involved in the Production of a Professional Videotape*: A reasonable assessment of all that it will take out of your time and your client's budget must be a major factor in your decision-making process from the outset.
3. *Work With a Team of Experienced Professionals*: Complicated videotapes such as the one used in this case study require the continued input of legal, medical, and telecommunication experts at every step of the process.
4. *Don't Feel Compelled to Use the Videotape at Trial*: As any experienced litigator knows, strategy and tactics for providing an optimal defense in complicated cases such as that discussed in this chapter may change constantly throughout a trial. Whether or not the videotape which you, your client, and however many others have so painstakingly produced is appropriate for admission into evidence may only be

ascertained once the courtroom drama begins to unfold. The propriety and timing of its presentation must be governed by the sound judgment of the experienced trial lawyer, in continuing consultation with his or her medical client.

8. Dementia and Trauma

Nathaniel Shafer, M.D.

Maurice Ravel was among the most important composers of the twentieth century. It is through his medical history that we have come to know more of him than about other musicians. The medical history of his later life is particularly interesting, due to a sudden, rapid decline in his intellectual and musical powers during his most productive years. We now recognize this decline to be a manifestation of a syndrome known as dementia or Alzheimer's disease. The medical evidence leaves little doubt that Ravel was stricken, quite suddenly, with dementia.

Ravel was born in the Pyrenees in 1875, and entered the Paris Conservatory in 1889. He later studied under Gabriel Fauré. Ravel and Debussy became representatives of the Impressionistic school, noted for their lyrical, rhythmic, yet economical musical styles. Ravel was an accomplished orchestrator and composer for the piano.

In 1931, at the age of 56, Ravel was completing two major piano works, *Concerto for the Left Hand* and the *G Major Concerto*. Months after finishing these pieces, he began to complain of increased fatique and lassitude—symptoms that were perhaps consistent with his chroic insomnia and hypochondriacal complaints. However, his creative energies suddenly decreased.

In October, 1932, Ravel was involved in a minor traffic accident in which he suffered facial cuts and bruises. Although there did not appear to be serious neurological sequellae, it was shortly after this event that his mental powers began to noticeably decline. His capacity to remember names, speak spontaneously, and write became impaired. These disabilities progressed rapidly during the following year. During his consultation with a noted French neurologist, Professor Alajouanine, it was observed that Ravel's ability to understand spoken words was superior to his ability to speak spontaneously or to write. Unfortunately, he also began to experience an inability to produce or comprehend musical sounds. His attempts at orchestral conducting failed, as he was no longer capable of the speech, coordination, and cognition required for such a task.

By 1934, he was no longer able to write script; letter-writing became laborious. The efforts of his friends to help him were futile. Gradually, his speech and intellectual functions declined further. By 1936, he was essentially mute and incapable of recognizing even his own music.

Following the automobile accident in October, 1932, Ravel composed virtually nothing other than two short songs for a movie project. He died in 1937.

Alzheimer's disease progresses to death in five to ten years. Like all dementias, it is characterized by memory defects, loss of orientation to time, shallowness of affect, progressive decrease in intellectual functions, and impairment of judgement. Motor functioning is invariably affected. Therefore, one can assume—given the history as outlined—that Ravel had this disease, which robbed him of his artistic gifts at the height of his creative years. Prior to his death, neurosurgical treatment was attempted, but the results and indications are far from clear. No autopsy was reported, for the family attempted to keep the details of his illness a private affair.

> Dementia means the deterioration in intellectual capacity. The condition is distinguished from mental retardation, in which subnormal intellectual ability has been lifelong, and may or may not be caused by brain injury; and from aphasia and Korsakoff's psychosis, in which specific intellectual skills (language and memory, respectively) have deteriorated without a proportial disturbance in other cognitive functions.[1]

Alzheimer originally described patients suffering from the disease as being aphasic, with paranoia and impaired memories.[2] Also noted were agraphia, paraphasia, and alexia. While the term "Alzheimer's disease" used to be applied to presenile dementia, it now applies to all cases of dementia.

POST-TRAUMATIC DEMENTIA

In 1928, Martland first drew attention to the problem of dementia following head injury.[3] He described the tendency for experienced boxers to become unsteady on their feet, to become forgetful, and to think and move more slowly than in their pre-boxing days. He reported that this condition was well known to fight fans and promoters, who referred to such a boxer as being "slugged nutty" or as "cutting paper dolls." The Germans used the term "soft pear" and, later, Millespaugh, in the United States, introduced the term, dementia pugilistica.[4]

Corsellis raised two concerns relating to head injury and post-traumatic dementia.[5] One was that a blow to the head may be followed by "progressive dementia of the Alzheimer type," and the other was the "possibility for irreversible damage caused by repeated blows to the head." The latter condition was clear-cut with professional boxers, where there were multiple head injuries that involved many episodes of unconsciousness and a clearly delineated picture of brain damage (dementia pugilistica). A 1969 survey focused on 224 ex-professional boxers who had been picked at random from the Register of the British Board of Boxing Control.[6] Of these, 17 percent exhibited an "easily recognized and relatively stereotyped syndrome of disturbed neurological function which variously affects the cerebellar, pyramidal, and extrapyramidal pathways, while on the psychiatric side . . . a variable degree of defective intellectual function, particularly of memory."

When there are few injuries (e.g., one head injury in an accident), subsequent signs of deterioration may be very slow, subtle, and insidious. Many might not become apparent for years, and one might think that such mental changes were part of the aging process. It is not surprising, therefore, that this condition was a matter of controversy for many years, especially when problems of litigation occurred concerning an automobile accident or on-the-job injury.

Corsellis et al. reported the case of a 50-year-old man who had been knocked unconscious while a passenger in a car.[7] He had been highly successful businessman but after the accicent—during which he was unconscious only for a few minutes—he deteriorated progressively, dying in a demented state several years later. He too was found to have been suffering from Alzheimer's disease. The question arose as to whether this was an extremely rare example of this condition that had been precipitated by trauma. Similarly, Miller, in reviewing the literature, remarked that such a sequence of events has almost always followed a minor injury.[8] He posited that such injuries simply brought attention to presenile dementia.

PATHOLOGIC STUDIES

The delay in the acceptance of the existence of this clinical syndrome may have been due to the paucity of neuropathological studies. Brains are often not made available on postmortem examination. Martland believed that the condition he had described was a result of scarring in the wake of petechial hemorrhages that had been scattered, particularly through the deeper parts of the cerebral hemispheres.[3] He admitted that he derived the idea from experiences with acute head injuries, but he had never had the opportunity to examine the brain of a boxer. He ended with a modest plea for neuropathologists to investigate the problem (which they began to do many years later). Hence, another paradox and dilemma: The syndrome was readily accepted in boxers suffering repeated blows to the head. There were some who claimed that one blow was not sufficient to cause the clinical picture of post-traumatic dementia. Yet, Martland's studies, in 1928, were done on patients who experienced single, acute head injuries.

In 1954, Brandenburg et al. described the findings of an ex-amateur boxing champion who had died in a demented state (Parkinsonian signs) at age 51.[9] The essential neuropathological features consisted of Alzheimer's disease with congophilic angiopathy. This was considered by Brandenburg to be a true case of dementia pugilistica, or post-traumatic dementia. Other investigators soon drew attention by discussing the abundance of Alzheimer's neurofibrillary tangles—but absence of neuritic plaques—in the brains of boxers that had been examined.[10,11]

Corsellis reported on twelve professional and three amateur boxers. All but three had Alzheimer's neurofibrillary tangles, and usually a rather substantial amount.[5] All but one had these tangles, to some extent, in the cerebral cortex. "As already pointed out, therefore, the one link with Alzheimer's disease is the intriguing tendency for neurofibrillary tangles to develop in remarkably large numbers, albeit in association with no, or very few, neuritic plaques."

Rudelli states: "Dementia pugilistica and rare cases of classic Alzheimer's disease following head injury suggest that trauma may also play a provocative role in neurofibrillary change. The ages and clinical descriptions, however, allow other interpretations.[12] A 38-year-old man died 16 years after substantial recovery from a single episode of severe head trauma. Pathologic study indicated that the clinical deterioration was due to classic Alzheimer's disease.

Spillane emphasized the frequency of chronic cerebral disorders in the elderly boxers.[13] He particularly stressed the symptoms of aggressiveness as being due to brain damage, and pointed out that, in four of his five cases, there was evidence of air pictures of structural anomalies in the septum pellucidum. He denied that these were due to mere coincidence or the effect of age and cerebral degeneration.

Corsellis[5] considered the neuropathological findings under four main headings:

1. Septal and hypothalamic anomalies,
2. Cerebellum,
3. Degeneration of substantia nigra, and
4. Regional occurrence of Alzheimer's neurofibrillary tangles.

The changes in the cerebellum were of particular interest. Here there was a frequently noticeable scarring of the folia in the region of the cerebellar tonsils. In addition, there was usually a marked reduction in the number of Purkinje cells on the undersurface of the cerebellar hemispheres. "This scarring appears to be the result of the repeated movement of the cerebellum against the foramen magnum in a way reminiscent of that seen by Lindenburg and Freytag in cases of acute cerebral trauma."[14]

In cases of severe dementia, with persistent vegetative state following brain injury, extensive degeneration of white matter is found at autopsy.[15,16] Thus, a variety of acute traumatic blows to the head may produce brain damage, leading to cognitive defects, confusion, memory loss, and the entire symptomology of dementia. Other changes that have been described include:

- septal tearing
- atrophy (particularly of the mamillary bodies)
- stretching of the floor of the hypothalamus
- tendency for the substantia nigra to become deficient in pigment
- gliosis of nerve cells.[5]

The extent of these changes will depend upon the severity and number of blows to the head.

SYMPTOMS AND DIAGNOSIS

The symptoms of dementia are as numerous as they are divergent. Clinical approach is difficult, due to varying signs and manifestations. Furthermore, there is evidence that severity of symptoms and clinical dysfunction correlate poorly with the severity of the disease process, as seen pathologically.[17]

The most common and easily detectable neurological-psychological disturbance following head trauma is post-traumatic amnesia. The patient may not remember what happened during the period of unconsciousness, or whether he or she was unconscious at all. It may be remembered as a brief period of confusion. Headaches and dizziness are common complaints. Irritability is not unusual. It may be difficult for the patient to concentrate or acquire new information. Recovery is not always complete, and some degree of memory disturbance may persist. However, while an important symptom of dementia is loss of recent memory, every normal, healthy individual has experienced the situation where he has just misplaced an object and cannot find it, or cannot remember if he took a pill that was prescribed by his physician.[18] The dividing line between what is normal and what is abnormal may not be clearly defined. The transition from old age to senile dementia, for example, is ordinarily gradual, and opinions as to when senility has set in are not always definitive.

Another problem arises when symptoms do not start immediately after the head injury, or when patients develop symptoms after an interval (sometimes as long as several years) of apparently normal intellectual functioning. In such cases, the following possibilities may be considered:

- The dementia is related to the trauma
- A new, coincidental illness has occurred
- The changes of normal aging may be magnified as a result of the traumatic effects.

Many of the signs and symptoms that occur during senile dementia may be seen in normal individuals. These include the following:

- A dislike of change
- Reduction in ambition and activity

- Tendency to become constricted, with self-centered interests
- Increased difficulty in comprehension
- Increase in time and effort necessary for the performance of familiar duties
- Increasing difficulty in adapting to new circumstances
- Lessened sympathy for new ideas and views
- Tendency to reminisce and repeat.

An individual may be diagnosed or considered as being senile or having senile dementia. Yet, to the inexperienced, he or she may appear to have moments of lucicity that will cause one to doubt the diagnosis. These experiences are not at all inconsistent with the diagnosis of senile dementia; once such a diagnosis has been made such occurrences should not change one's evaluation of the condition. In general, in instances of senile dementia due to Alzheimer's disease, there are no well-defined remissions. They are not to be expected, and only if they occur should one question the diagnosis. Dementia due to Alzheimer's disease tends to be progressive.[19]

A list of symptoms of dementia includes the following:

1. Amnesia
2. Reduced learning
3. Reduced retention and recall of events
4. Confabulation
5. Disturbances of attention and concentration
6. Lack of initiative and spontaneity; reduced stock of ideas
7. Impoverishment of thoughts and associations; increased reactivity
8. Extreme selectiveness of stimuli
9. Inability to survery, integrate, and analyze information
10. Tendency toward catastrophic reactions
11. Disturbances of consciousness (dozing off, wakefulness)
12. Disorientation; affective disturbances; emotional shallowness; reduction in general interest and in the awareness of own illness
13. Euphoria; affective liability
14. Increased irritability; suspicious and paranoid tendencies
15. Disturbances of language; aphasia; agnosia; inability to understand nonverbal symbols
16. Apraxia
17. Incapacity for carrying out purposeful movements; diminished energy and enthusiasm
18. Anxiety; diminished creativity; self-concern; depression; outbursts of anger; delayed recall
19. Slowed speech; impaired understanding; neglect of personal appearance; disorientation as to time and place; trouble following directions; unsteady gait; rocky movements of the trunk and neck

20. Inappropriate gestures of the hands; facial grimaces; tremors; tendency to sit or stand in a bent position
21. Rigidity of limbs; licking or pursing of lips
22. Repetition in movement or speech.[20]

The earliest symptoms of dementia or brain damage can pass almost unrecognized, and may be very subtle at the beginning, appearing only as disturbances in the patient's solving of problems, grasp of situations, and agility of thought. He or she may carry out the daily routine at home and work adequately, but becomes more inefficient, failing in the tasks that are more demanding or require special skills. This author has seen patients suffering head injuries who have appeared normal in the hospital and while under his care. They appeared normal to their spouses also, but, upon returning to work, could not perform the duties they were accustomed to performing before the head injury.

A physician suffering from dementia may thus be able to manage the easier cases and those more familiar to him, but is less adept at diagnosing and prescribing for the new and more difficult ones. A teacher may have to make an unusual effort, or spend more time on a routine lesson or lecture; he or she may be puzzled by questions from students that go beyond the prepared material.

Many of the symptoms of depression—or the changes seen with dementia—may be hard to distinguish from fatigue or boredom. Many times, appreciation of patients' symptoms will not come until after a full examination. Relatives may not even be aware of the mental changes; these may be first reported by one's boss or supervisor. Professional, managerial, or skilled workers are more quickly brought in for help than are individuals in unskilled occupations. One 42-year-old executive was brought to this author for help, though nothing could be found mentally or physically wrong with him. However, it was this patient's fellow workers who insisted that the man's skills had fallen off abruptly. After a complete work-up, a brain tumor was found, and the patient was cured.

It should be stressed that, as a rule, the patient with dementia has little or no realization of these changes in himself. As the condition progresses, there is a loss of almost all intellectual faculties. It has been suggested that the failure of intellectual function serves as a compensation for the meanness of the diseases—that it spares the patient from knowing what has happened to him.

In the early stages of dementia, the patient may be unable to use words with facility; he will depend on clichés and habitual forms of expression. This facade of customary manners, however, cannot hide the deficits in mental capacity, if in examination talk is carried beyond casual interchange to test memory, orientation, and grasp of situations and concepts.

Wells states: "Defects in orientation, memory, intellectual functioning, judgement, and affectivity are stressed in the usual account of the symptomatology of dementia. These classic features may indeed dominate the clinical picture, but then to focus exclusively on these symptoms is to emphasize the end states of the dementing process.''[17] Thus, it is not difficult to recognize and notice intellectual impairment in individuals late in the course of the cerebral disease.

The more taxing problem lies in the recognition of the intellectual impairment early, when it is slight, perhaps potentially reversible, but perhaps leading to impaired perception if not caught in time. Testing a patient's cognitive functioning—part of every neurologic examination—may accomplish this. It is customary to test the following:

1. Orientation to time, place, and people
2. Language skills, asking the patient to name common objects and respond to demands
3. Fund of knowledge, such as the names of presidents and capital cities
4. Recent memory, by setting three objects to be remembered for 5, 10, and 30 minutes
5. Attention span, by asking for a serial substraction of seven from one hundred, or any other arithmetical tests requiring ''carrying over''
6. Abstract reasoning power, by asking for definitions of proverbs, or the similarity of words such as apple, orange, ear, eye
7. Constructional capacity, by asking the patient to draw a simple object such as a clock, or to copy an abstract.

The results of these tests must be interpreted in the light of other information about the patient. If the patient was a gifted professional person, in whom a decline in judgement and increasing forgetfulness has been noted, the discovery that he or she cannot hold three words in mind for five minutes and that he or she interprets problems clumsily provides compelling evidence that he or she is suffering from a disturbance of intellectual power. On the other hand, if the person was not particularly gifted, or was poorly educated, the results of these tests are interpreted accordingly. It should be appreciated, however, that not all intellectual functions are affected to an equal degree, or need be affected individually, in dementia.

Testing for recent memory and functional capacity is most useful, and efficiency here is easy to document. In matters of medical-legal importance, documentation review of the patient's record may be necessary to establish the presence of dementia or impaired judgement, as in the matter of the probate of a will. The records may speak forthrightly (or not at all) about the presence of confusion. The absence of such statements in records does not indicate the endorsement of mental competence, especially when the patient is in a general hospital. In such cases, the main problem may be the treatment of an acute coronary or a bleeding episode, in which case the physician and nurses of record will be equipped to handle the emergency medical problems. However, should the records indicate the presence of severe medical diseases, such as shock, heart failure, liver failure, or other conditions such as hepatic encephalopathy, uremia, or anemia, which commonly affect cognitive function, one can be certain that this type of patient can be responsible for none of his acts.

CASE REPORT

A 78-year-old man suffered shock for a duration of one hour, with a blood pressure of 0. There was extensive arteriosclerosis. This person most definitely suffered cerebral, cardiac, and renal anoxia as result of this shock. After receiving multiple transfusions, he went on to develop hepatitis and had an elevated serum ammonia, which was life-threatening. He was in and out of a somnolent and comatose state and, during one period of alertness, a will was given to him to sign. It was not difficult to establish that this patient was not intellectually or cognitively competent. The records documented extensive vascular disease, the presence of heart failure, uremia, liver disease, and shock. In addition, the patient had been on multiple drugs, which impaired cognition.

UNDERLYING AND REVERSIBLE CAUSES

Where dementia has a specific underlying cause, one may expect a reversal of symptoms. Yet, where there is an associated process of senility, or where brain damage has occurred, the organic dementia generally persists. Dementia should never be attributed to simply growing old, as senile dementia may also be a sign or symptom of a serious and potentially fatal disease (brain tumor, liver failure, respiratory failure, or kidney failure). Treatment of hypothyroidism, pernicious anemia, and other endocrine abnormalities may produce a complete reversal of the organic dementia. Dementia, in some cases, may be due to a chronic meningitis or encephalitis. This can only be diagosed by a spinal tap, which will be obtained only when it is suspected that there is such an underlying cause.

While depression maybe an early symptom of dementia, it is nonetheless important to ascertain whether depression is a cause of a patient's symptoms of confusion and slowed speech. Depression may mimic the entire clinical picture of Alzheimer's disease, or dementia. This differentiation is crucial, since depression is quite treatable. Information about recent losses of relatives, friends, status, and funds should be sought in the history. Symptoms of insomnia and hypochondriasis should also be sought, as these may occur in dementia. Depression may occur without a provocative cause.

It is helpful to ask the older patient to bring his medications to the office so that the physician can see what is being taken. Untoward reactions to barbiturates, reserpine, alcohol, and sedatives should be considered as a possible cause of depression. The anticholinergic side effects of both the antidepressants and antipsychotics include blurred vision, dryness of the mouth, constipation, urinary retention, and arrhythmias. One may see symptoms of delerium such as mental clouding, confusion, inability to pay attention, disorientation, speech blockade, delusions, agitation, and convulsions. The elderly—especially the demented elderly or those on drugs that may interact with the antipsychotics—are particularly prone to develop a delerium.

Hearing-impaired (not deaf) individuals also not uncommonly suffer from a paranoidlike condition, with ideas of reference. Moreover, fifteen percent of myocardial infarctions in the elderly present with a mental-status change, without chest pain.

DISCUSSION

As of 1950, 8 percent—12.3 million—of the population in the United States was over 55 years of age. By 1978, this figure rose to 11 percent—22 million people. It is estimated that by the year 2030 those over the age of 65 will constitute between 17 and 20 percent of the population (51 million). The costs of caring for demented patients are expected to soar from the 1978 figure of $12 billion per annum to $30 billion in 2030. The toll that dementia takes on the patient is enormous, and the effect it has on their families is overwhelming. "Dementia is one of the greatest problems facing modern society, and yet is one that seems little appreciated. The condition affects one person in every six over the age of 65. Those affected survive only one-third as long as healthy people of the same age and sex."[21]

Each year, head injuries produce permanent cognitive and behavioral deficits in a large number of individuals.[22] "Head injury can engender persistent neuropsychological and psychiatric damage that ranges from subtle disturbances in perception, information processing, language, memory, personality, or mood, to severe intellectual and emotional disturbance, or even chronic vegetative states."[23] The mental changes in the patient following head injury—(personality and memory deficits)—tend to cause families more difficulty than does physical disability.[24, 25]

Guilleminault et al. have studied patients complaining of excessive daytime sleeping (EDS) related to significant head trauma.[26] They have found that objectively confirmed post-traumatic EDS can be a significant problem, leading in some cases to long-term disability. It was concluded that the severity of the initial head trauma, judged by the duration of the initial coma, correlated with the severity of the long-term subjective EDS complaints.

"Fifty percent of patients with significant head trauma die at the scene of the accident or within 48 hours of admission to the hospital. Appoximately 10 percent of all head-injured patients who survive the head trauma require prolonged hospitalization for temporary or permanent neurological disability."[27]

"A hundred consecutive patients, in whom head injury had been associated with post-traumatic amnesia of more than 24-hours duration, had been seen. . . . and the 92 survivors were subsequently reexamined. Of the 92, ten showed some degree of dementia . . . "[28]

" . . . All surviving cases except one (26 persons) in a population of severe traumatic brain injuries with an initial period of unconsciousness of one week or more, examined at least two years after the injury, show (in general) a clinically observable reduction in 'capacity' (memory, learning, concentration) as well as psychomotor and energy. A correlation had been found between these reactions and the length of post-traumatic amnesia time. The matched control group chosen from a clientele of slight mental cases clearly differentiates from the brain injury groups in regard to these functions . . . "[29]

"The picture of severe post-traumatic dementia, with global disorganization of intellect, usually accompanied by striking neurological disablement, is well known . . . "[30] "(It) usually presents with much the same diverse constellation of symptoms as dementia produced from any other cause."[31]

CASE REPORT

"A 22-year-old involved in car accident suffered a head injury in December, 1963, resulting in loss of consciousness and left frontotemporal skull fracture. Bilateral burr holes show small, acute subdural hemorrhages. Progressive coma and pupillary fluctuation led to evacuation of a left temporal hematoma and surrounding contused brain. Patient left the hospital after four weeks with moderate dysphasia, anterograde and retrograde amnesia, and impaired judgement and abstract thinking. The following 18 months saw improvement (return to job, etc.). Patient received phenytoin sodium b/c, and EEG showed left temporal sharp and slow waves. July 1970—bilateral-temporal cranioplasty performed; 1971—behavioral changes: impulsive outbursts, absenteeism; 1973—psych. testing showing regression of reading level to grade 1 from grade 3, evidence of apraxia and occasional tremor in both arms; 1974—loss of job. Experiences urinary incontinence."[12]

APPENDIX: SYMPTOMS OF DEMENTIA

Early signs:

1. Spending more time in work to achieve less results
2. Little less articulate in expressing views
3. Forgetting what one has said, or nature of conversation
4. Diminished energy and enthusiasm
5. Loss of interest and concern for vocation, family, social activity
6. Increased anxiety
7. Less interest in goals and achievements
8. Diminished creativity
9. Less incentive to stick to a task
10. Difficulty concentrating
11. Greater annoyance at failures, frustrations, changes
12. Increased absorption with oneself and own problems
13. Difficulty making plans

14. Inability to decide where to go on vacation
15. Difficulty dealing with new situations, initiating activity
16. Avoiding choices in decisions
17. Unreliability in calculations
18. Lowered motivation
19. Appropriate dress and personal cleanliness ignored
20. No interest in the opinion of others
21. Personal warmth and concern for others disappearing*
22. Apathy; blunting of all feelings, eliciting brief responses
23. Defective recent memory

Later signs:

24. Calculations impossible
25. Perception is blurred and distorted
26. Incontinence
27. Stupor
28. Coma
29. Sleeping all day, difficult to arouse at times.

*This is often thought to represent hostility, leading to family squabbles which, actually, can be the cause of disinheritence—leaving money not to children who had been loved for a lifetime, and who cared for their parent, but to a foundation. This should be taken as evidence of dementia—that an elderly parent, who in not leaving his or her money to the children and grandchildren, but to people he or she does not know, has become gullible.

The author gratefully acknowledges the assistance of Garry Kitay in the preparation of this manuscript.

REFERENCES

1. McHugh, P.R. "Dementia," in *Textbook of Medicine*, Beeson, P.B., McDermott, W., eds. Philadelphia. W. B. Saunders Co., 1975, 558.

2. Alzheimer, A., "A unique illness involving the cerebral cortex," in *Neurologic Classics in Modern Translation*, Rottenbert, D.A. and Hochberg, F.H., eds. New York, Haffner Press, 1977, 41–43.

3. Martland, H.S., "Punch drunk." *JAMA* 1928; 91:1103–1107.

4. Millespaugh, J.A., "Dementia pugilistica." *U.S. Naval Medical Bulletin*, 1937; 35:297–303.

5. Corosellis, J.A.N., "Post-traumatic dementia," in *Aging*, Katzman R., Terry R.D., and Bick K.L., eds. New York: Raven Press, 1978, 125.

6. Roberts, A.H., "Brain damage in boxers. A study of prevalence of traumatic encephalopathy among ex-professional boxers." London: Pitman, 1969.

7. Corsellis J.A.N., et al, "Observations on the pathology of insidious dementia following head injury." *J. Ment. Sci.*, 1959; 105:714–20.

8. Miller, H., "Mental after-effects of head injury." *Proc. R. Soc. Med.*, 1966; 59:257–61.

9. Brandenburg, W., and Hallerrorden, J., "Dementia Pugilistica Mitanatomischen Befund." *Virchows Arch* 1964; 325:680–709.

10. Graham, H., and Ule, G., Beitrag zur kenntinis dere chronischen cerebralen krankheit spilder der boxern. *Psychiatr. Neurol.*, 1957; 134:261–83.

11. Mortimer, J.A., French, L.R., Hutten, J.T., and Schuman, L.M., "Head injury as a risk factor for Alzheimer's disease." *Neurology*, 1985; 35(2):264–67.

12. Rudelli, R., Strom, J., Welch, P.T., et al., "Post-traumatic premature Alzheimer's disease." *Arch. Neurol.*, 1982; 39:570.

13. Spillane J.D., "Five boxers." *Br. Med. J.*, 1962; 2:1205–1210.

14. Lindenburgh, R., and Freytag, L., "The mechanism of cerebral contusions." *Arch. Path.*, 1960; 69:440–69.

15. Jellinger, K., and Seidelberger, F., "Protracted and post-traumatic encephalopathy." *J. Neurol. Sci.*, 1970; 10:51–94.

16. Courville, C.D., "The mechanism of cou-contrecoup injury to the brain." *Bull Los Angeles Neurol. Sci.*, 1950; 15:72–86.

17. Wells, C.E., "The symptoms and behavioral manifestations of dementia," in *Dementia*, Wells, C.E., ed. Philadelphia: F. A. Davis Co., 1971; pp. 1–12.

18. Kolb, L.C., *Modern Clinical Psychiatry*. Philadelphia: W. B. Saunders Co., 1977; 158–59.

19. *Ibid*, 330–31.

20. Ludwig, A.M., *Principles of Clinical Psychology*. New York: The Free Press, 1980, 238–44.

21. Mortimer, J.A., Hepburn, K. and Meletta, G.J., "Alzheimer's disease: the intersection of diagnosis, research and long-term care." *Bull. N.Y. Acad. Med.*, 1985; 61:331–42.

22. Cummings, J.L., and Benson, D.F., *Dementia*. Boston: Butterworths, 1983, p. 249.

23. Kwentud, J.A., Hart, R.P., Peck, E.T., Kirnstein, S., "Psychiatric complications of closed head trauma." *Psychosomatics*, 1985; 26(1):8–13.

24. Bond, M.R., "Assessment of the psychological outcome after severe head injury." *Ciba Foundation Symposium*, 1975; 34:141–153.

25. Brooks D.N., and Aughton, M.E., "Psychological consequences of blunt-head injury." *Int. Rehabil. Med.*, 1979: 1:160–65.

26. Guilleminault, C., Faull, K.F., Miles, L., and Van den Hoed, J., "Post-traumatic excessive daytime sleepiness: a review of twenty patients." *Neurology*, 1983; 33:1584–89.

27. Alexander, N.P., "Traumatic Brain Injury," in *Psychiatric Aspects of Neurological Disease*, Binson D.F., and Blumer, D., eds. vol. 2. New York: Grune and Stratton, 1982, 249–58.

28. Miller, H., and Stern, G., "The long-term prognosis of severe head injury." *Lancet*, 1965; 1:225–29.

29. Norrman, B., and Svahn, K., "A follow-up study of severe brain injuries." *Acta. Psych. Scan.*, 1961; 37:236–264.

30. Lishiman, W.H., "The psychiatric sequelae of head injury." *Psychol. Med.*, 1973; 3:304–318.
31. Parker, N., "Post-traumatic dementia." *Proc. Aust. Assoc. Neurol.*, 1969; 16:39–44.

9. Beyond the Right to Life—The Right to Health

Sharon M. Camissa, Esquire and Natalie Ziontz, Esquire

INTRODUCTION

In 1983, a doctor in Baltimore, Maryland petitioned a court to take custody of an unborn fetus and order its mother, a habitual drug user, to undergo drug rehabilitation treatment. The doctor testified that the mother's drug habits endangered the life and well-being of the fetus and could cause debilitating birth defects.[1]

As this case suggests, conflict between the rights of a pregnant woman and the rights of the fetus is emerging as a medical, legal, and ethical problem. This chapter explores the tension between a pregnant woman's right to do as she wishes with her own body, and the right of a fetus to a healthy existence once the mother has decided to carry the pregnancy to term.

Under existing law, a state must have a compelling interest[2] in protecting a fetus before it can impinge on an individual's privacy rights.[3] Thus, a state is constitutionally limited in its ability to protect an unborn child.[4]

During the past two decades, medical researchers have accumulated considerable knowledge of the human fetus and its environment.[5] They now know that a mother's conduct affects the fetus.[6] This paper would argue that, in some situations, the fetus' rights prevent a mother from harming it, and also draws attention to possible authorities under which states could intervene on its behalf.

Section I presents medical evidence relating to the likelihood and severity of harm done to a fetus through actions by its mother. Section II is a historical survey of the fetus' legal rights. Section III discusses the conflict between the constitutional rights of a woman and those of a fetus. Section IV proposes a statutory amendment as a solution to the conflict. A proposed amendment to an existing California statute illustrates this solution. Section V discusses the future status of a woman's right to privacy in light of a changing Supreme Court.

I. MEDICAL ADVANCES IN FETAL CARE

Advances in medical technology raise important questions about the legal relationship between a mother and her fetus. Until recently, scientists knew little about the fetus' intrauterine environment.[7] However, in the last two decades, researchers have learned a great deal about prenatal life.[8] This knowledge has given the fetus the status of a separate patient, entitling it to separate care and treatment.[9]

A mother may jeopardize the life or health of the fetus by refusing treatment for herself that would benefit the fetus. Using new medical discoveries, physicians can now protect a fetus from disabilities that were once permanent or fatal.[10] These procedures, however, depend on the cooperation of the mother; physicians are only able to reach the fetus through her body. Advancements in fetal care increase the likelihood of situations in which a mother's right to refuse treatment will conflict with the fetus' need for it.[11]

The increased frequency of substance abuse in the United States[12] has increased the likelihood of conflict between mothers' and fetuses' rights.[13] Alcohol and drugs threaten damage to a developing fetus.[14] For example, the use of cocaine[15] or heroin during pregnancy adversely affects a developing fetus.[16] Despite the illegality of these drugs, their use is commonplace.[17] Under current laws, fetuses are entitled to protection from the detrimental effects of drugs, and in this context there would appear to be no significant difference between illegal and legal drugs.

Alcohol, a legal substance, is even more dangerous to a developing fetus.[18] Its prevalence, legality, and availability actually increase its potential danger.[19] Physicians have long recognized the relationship between birth defects and alcohol use during pregnancy.[20] However, medical researchers did not discover a specific pattern of alcohol-related malformations until 1968.[21] In 1973, researchers coined the term "fetal alcohol syndrome" to refer to a pattern of altered growth in infants who had been exposed to large amounts of alcohol before birth.[22] In recent years, research has confirmed the risk of adverse effects to infants born to alcoholic mothers.[23] Infants with this disorder suffer from many different kinds of abnormalities.[24] Unlike the symptoms of infant drug withdrawal, these symptoms do not disappear with age.[25] The affected infant must live with these abnormalities for life.[26] Thus, the fetus needs protection from maternal substance abuse.

A woman has a constitutionally protected right to abort a fetus during the early stages of her pregnancy.[27] This right, however, does not necessarily give her the right to abuse the fetus once she has decided to carry it to term.[28] A father or an interested state agency might seek to compel an unwilling mother to undergo treatment for drug or alcohol addiction for the fetus' benefit. The following sections discuss authorities under which they could seek this compulsion.

II. FETAL PROTECTION—A HISTORICAL PERSPECTIVE AND A PRESENT APPLICATION

Unborn fetuses have long received legal protection. However, lawmakers may assign fetal rights more or less importance depending on the other interests at play.

In early English common law, the fetus had certain limited property rights from the time of conception.[29] However, many property rights of the unborn were vested only when the child was born alive.[30] Although this live birth requirement still persists today, legislatures have acted to protect the inheritance rights of the unborn.[31]

Some state courts and legislatures also interpret criminal statutes to protect fetal rights. The general penal code sections that protect living persons from murder or physical abuse may protect the unborn as well. For example, in *Keeler v. Superior Court*[32] the California Supreme Court held that a viable fetus was not a "person" within the meaning of the state's homicide statute.[33] In respose to *Keeler*, the California legislature amended the homicide statute to make it unlawful to kill a human being "or fetus" regardless of age.[34]

California Penal code section 270,[35] also interpreted to protect a fetus, makes it a misdemeanor for a father to willfully fail to support his minor child.[36] Michigan has extended fetal protection even further by upholding a criminal indictment for child abuse when a woman gave birth to a heroin-addicted infant.[37]

Tort law also provides increasing protection for fetuses.[38] For example, as early as 1946 a court recognized the right of a fetus, born alive, to sue for prenatal injuries.[39] This court held that only fetuses viable at the time of injury could obtain relief. Some courts, however, have extended this protection to include fetuses injured before viability.[40] Courts in some states have also allowed plaintiffs to recover tort damages for the wrongful death of a fetus. California, along with a number of other jurisdictions, still refuses to allow a stillborn fetus to be the subject of a wrongful death suit.[41] However, a substantial number of states, led by Minnesota, now allow recovery for prenatal death under wrongful death statutes.[42]

While courts are increasingly sympathetic to the plight of the fetus and are willing to interpret statutes as including protection and recompense for it, the fetus needs more solid protection. This paper proposes statutory reform or, alternatively, clearly mandated statutory interpretation of relevant statutes for the protection of substance-abused fetuses. Statutory reform allowing protection of an endangered fetus would provide uniformity and consistency in the protection of fetal rights. These reforms would be consistent with the constitutional framework for balancing the rights of mother and fetus mandated in *Roe v. Wade*.[43] According to *Roe*, the state's ability to protect the fetus is limited by the woman's privacy right.[44]

The next section gives an overview of the right to privacy. It then discusses the impact of recent cases on the conflicting rights of mother and fetus.

III. THE DEVELOPMENT OF CONFLICTING RIGHTS—THE RIGHT TO PRIVACY AND THE RIGHT TO REFUSE TREATMENT VERSUS THE RIGHT TO LIFE

A. The Right to Privacy

The landmark decision recognizing a woman's right to privacy and personal autonomy was *Roe v. Wade*.[45] However, *Roe* was not the first case to establish an individual's right to privacy. The United States Supreme Court first recognized a fundamental constitutional right to privacy in *Griswold v. Connecticut*.[46] Subsequent cases both extend and limit *Griswold*.[47]

Roe extended the privacy right to include the right to terminate a pregnancy. In *Roe*, the Court considered the constitutionality of Texas statutes that criminalized abortion at any time during pregnancy unless necessary to save the mother's life.[48] The Court held that the statutes violated due process.[49] The Court also expressly extended the right to privacy, including in it a woman's decision to have an abortion.[50] However, the Court qualified the woman's right to privacy, holding that a compelling state interest could limit the breadth of this right.[51]

Roe protects a woman's right to privacy by expressly allowing her to choose to abort during the first part of her pregnancy. A woman's right to abort is absolute for the first twelve weeks of pregnancy. The state may not regulate abortion during this first trimester.[52] In the second trimester of pregnancy, the state may regulate abortion, but only if the regulation is reasonably related to maternal health.[53] In the third trimester, the state can prohibit abortions to preserve the potential life of the fetus.[54] the Court held that the woman's right to privacy outweighs the fetus' right to life, until the fetus is "potentially able to live outside the mother's womb, albeit with artificial aid."[55]

In later cases, the Court tried to clarify and explain its decision in *Roe*. These cases focused on the critical issue of viability. Viability is the point when a fetus is potentially able to live independently of its mother.[56] Physicians find it difficult to determine when a fetus is viable, because of the multiple considerations.[57] Although the *Roe* Court used viability as its dividing line, it recognized that individual physicians must determine viability on a case-by-case basis.[58]

In 1976, the Supreme Court restated its opinion that physicians must determine viability case-by-case.[59] In *Planned Parenthood of Central Missouri v. Danforth*[60] the petitioner questioned a statute defining viability as "that stage in fetal development when the life of the unborn child may be continued indefinitely outside the womb."[61] The Court held that the questioned statute preserved the necessary flexibility of the viability concept.[62]

Three years later, the Court, in *Coalutti v. Franklin*, invalidated a statute for vagueness on the viability issue.[63] The Court held that a physician could not be criminally liable for a good-faith error in assessing viability.[64] Thus, the Court upheld viability as the point when fetal rights attach.

In *Akron v. Akron Center for Reproductive Health, Inc.*, the Court invalidated several provisions in the state's abortion statute regulating abortions during the second trimester.[65] The majority recognized that, since *Roe* hd been decided, abortions had become safer later into pregnancy and that fetuses became viable earlier in pregnancy, thereby blurring an already obscure line.[66] However, the majority retained the trimester approach as the legal framework for limiting a state's authority to regulate abortions.[67]

Although the viability of a fetus is not easy to determine, it is the most appropriate point at which fetal rights should attach.[68] Viability is a better point than birth because the differences between a viable fetus and a newborn are insignificant.[69] Although a newborn has a greater chance of survival than a viable fetus, chances of survival for a viable fetus are increasing with each advance in perinatal care.[70] Thus, the differences between a viable fetus and a newborn are diminishing.

Viability is a convenient starting point at which to recognize fetal rights. It is the moment in development when the fetus' chances of becoming a contributing member of society are greatly enhanced.[71] However, in application, the viability framework has many difficulties.[72] One of the biggest difficulties is determining when a fetus has become viable. A fine line divides viable and nonviable fetuses.

Fortunately, the difficulties arising from the viability concept are not insurmountable.[73]

Viability is the most desirable point for the attachment of fetal rights that can override a mother's right to an abortion. However, the right to an abortion is only one derivative of the right to privacy. The next section discusses another derivative of the right to privacy, the right to refuse treatment, and its impact on fetal rights.

B. The Right to Refuse Treatment

The right to refuse treatment is an outgrowth of the right of privacy. However, the cases are unclear in specifying when courts first recognized it as a constitutionally protected right. The Constitution does not expressly grant this right,[74] however, the right to refuse treatment is clearly rooted in the common law.[75] Courts recognize that a competent adult has the constitutional right to refuse life-saving treatment.[76] The right to refuse treatment, like the right to choose whether or not to have an abortion, is qualified: a compelling state interest may override this right.[77]

In deciding whether or not a compelling state interest exists, courts generally consider two factors. The state may have a compelling interest in the preservation of an adult life if the patient has a dependent minor child.[78] In such a case, a hospital, physician, or other interested party would petition a court to override the patient's right to refuse life-saving medical care, and order treatment. Under these circumstances, the court could compel treatment.[79] Another compelling state interest arises when a patient's refusal of treatment would result in a risk to others.[80] Interested parties could petition the court for authority to compel treatment.

However, an individual's right to refuse treatment is more complex when the individual is a pregnant woman. If courts are willing to treat a viable fetus like a dependent minor, its mother can be compelled to undergo treatment to save her own life.[81]

In *Raleigh Fitkin–Paul Morgan Memorial Hospital v. Anderson*, the New Jersey Supreme Court ordered a pregnant woman in her third trimeter to have a blood transfusion, creating a conflict with her religious beliefs.[82] The court summarily stated that the fetus was entitled to legal protection.[83] Although *Anderson* was decided before *Roe*, the decision fits into the *Roe* framework regarding intrusion on a mother's privacy right. The *Roe* decision designated viability as the point at which state intervention is permissible.[84] In *Anderson* the court imposed treatment on a woman for the benefit of a viable fetus. This suggests that the state may be able to force a drug- or alcohol-addicted woman to undergo treatment if she is carrying a viable fetus.

A fetus is also an "other" at risk when its mother refuses life-saving treatment. Therefore, a woman whose refusal of treatment puts her fetus at risk should be ordered to submit to treatment.[85] Following this analysis, an alcoholic or drug addicted woman who was endangering the life of her fetus could be compelled to undergo treatment. However, a court must be willing to interpret "other" in this context to include a fetus; and no court has yet done this. This interpretation may also conflict with the *Roe* decision if an interested party seeks treatment before the fetus is viable.

C. Recognition of a Viable Fetus' Right to a Healthy Existence

Although courts have consistently upheld an individual's right to privacy and right to refuse treatment, recent cases severely limit these rights when the patient is a pregnant woman. *Jefferson v. Griffin Spaulding County Hospital Authority* examined the conflict between a viable fetus' right to life and a mother's right to privacy and to refuse medical treatment.[86] The hospital sued to compel a woman in her third trimester of pregnancy to submit to a cesarean section. A physician diagnosed the woman as having *placenta previa*, a condition occurring when the placenta blocks the birth canal. Physicians believed the fetus had a ninety-nine-percent chance of dying during natural childbirth.[87] They predicted a fifty-percent chance of survival for the mother without intervention.[88] The hospital petitioned the trial court for an order compelling the woman to have surgery. The court held that the state's abortion statute protected the viable fetus, and granted the order.[89] The court went further and allowed an appropriate state agency to petition the court to compel the woman to submit to the surgery before the onset of labor.[90]

The Department of Family and Child Services petitioned the Juvenile Court of Butts County, Georgia, for temporary custody of the fetus, and for an order compelling Mrs. Jefferson to undergo a cesarean. The court found that the fetus was a "deprivied child" under the state's neglect and dependency statutes.[91] The court awarded temporary custody to the county authority.[92] Mrs. Jefferson and her husband filed a motion to stay the order compelling surgery. Balancing the fetus' right to life against the mother's right to privacy, the Georgia Supreme Court denied the motion and affirmed the lower court's decision.[93]

The Jefferson court relied on *Roe* for the proposition that the state had a compelling interest in the life of a viable fetus. This interest permitted intrusion on the mother's constitutionally protected rights. This, however, was state intrusion far beyond that allowed in *Roe*.[94]

The *Jefferson* court also extended fetal protection by granting custody of the fetus to a county authority. This was more than a limitation on the mother's rights. By giving the state complete decision-making authority over medical treatment for the mother and fetus, the court prospectively denied the mother's right to refuse treatment during the remainder of her pregnancy.[95] *Jefferson* was the first appellate decision allowing a court's exercise of authority over a fetus.[96]

In *Taft v. Taft*, the Supreme Judicial Court of Massachusetts *in dictum* showed a willingness to extend fetal rights.[97] In *Taft*, a husband sued his pregnant wife to compel her to undergo surgery that would help her maintain the pregnancy. Without surgery, the mother would probably have miscarried.[98] The trial court gave the husband authority to consent to the surgery, even though the fetus was not yet viable. The Supreme Judicial Court of Massachusetts vacated the judgment. The court found no case law supporting mandatory surgery to save a pre-viable fetus.[99] However, the court suggested *in dictum* that some circumstances may compel restriction of a person's right to privacy on behalf of a pre-viable fetus.[100]

Jefferson and *Taft* suggest that the state may, in some circumstances, compel treatment for the benefit of the fetus.[101] The argument used in *Jefferson* could apply to situations involving a pregnant addict. In light of the fetal dangers, a court may order a pregnant woman to refrain from abusing her body to protect the unborn child. Courts may apply the *Jefferson* rationale to these situations as long as the fetus is viable. However, support for the imposition of treatment on a pre-viable fetus is scanty.[102]

Jefferson elucidates the possible solutions to a conflict between the rights of a mother and those of her fetus. It extends the *Roe* fetal protections to establish a pregnant woman's affirmative duty to take necessary steps to insure the birth and health of her fetus.[103] Imposition of this duty has profound implications on the rights of pregnant women; it diminishes the rights of women to make decisions about their bodies.[104]

Jefferson and the *Taft* dictum are only two state court opinions sanctioning state interference on a woman's rights to benefit her fetus. The *Jefferson* decision, however, does not offend the constitution. *Roe* allows a state to infringe on a woman's privacy right for the benefit of a viable fetus.[105] The *Jefferson* court ordered treatment on a woman carrying a viable fetus. Other courts may follow *Jefferson* because of its constitutional soundness. However, some courts may be reluctant to impose treatment on a pregnant woman without authorization from the United States Supreme Court. Therefore, a legislative solution is needed to insure protections for both mother and fetus and consistency among jurisdictions.

The final section of this Chapter proposes a legislative amendment, or, alternatively, judicial guidelines for deciding conflicts between the rights of a woman and those of her unborn child.

III. RESOLUTION OF THE CONFLICT

As the foregoing discussion indicates, a simple resolution of the conflict of rights between a woman and her fetus is unlikely. Those who jealously guard the individual's personal freedoms may espouse the position that no one ever has a right to invade the privacy of a pregnant woman, even to protect the fetus. This position, however, is not supported in the law.[106] Another position, not discussed in this chapter, focuses on the absolute right of the fetus to a healthy birth.[107] Commentators and case law have rejected this absolutist position as well.[108] Therefore, those who attempt to resolve these delicate questions must balance the rights of mother and unborn child in an attempt to protect the rights of each. The authors propose statutory reform as a method of achieving this delicate balance of rights.

A. Proposed Legislation

Legislators in many states have interpreted existing laws to protect fetuses.[109] A state's neglect and dependency statutes can provide complete and specific protection for the fetus while safeguarding the mother's right to personal autonomy. For example, California Welfare and Institutions Code, Section 300, protects endangered minors by making them dependent children of the state.[110] The authors propose legislation to amend state neglect and dependency statutes to include protections for viable fetuses. The California statute will serve as an example. An amendment to the California statute would read, in pertinent part: "Any *living* person under the age of 18 years, *or any unborn viable fetus* who comes within any of the following descriptions is within the jurisdiction of the juvenile court, whch may adjudge such person to be a dependent child of the court: . . . "[111] This section, if so amended, would safeguard the health of an abused fetus without the threat of punishment for the mother.[112] All the procedural safeguards required by Section 300 would also be required when applied to an unborn child.[113]

This amendment would be immune from constitutional attack if applied within the boundaries of *Roe*. For example, consider the situation presented in the beginning of this chapter. A physician becomes aware that a pregnant patient is addicted to drugs or alcohol. Under *Roe*, during the first trimester, the private physician could counsel the patient against the use of harmful substances, but courts would not allow state interference or compulsion.[114] During the second trimester, when the fetus is not yet viable, Roe continues to prohibit state intervention on behalf of the fetus.[115] Therefore, a physician could recommend counseling or, in extreme cases, abortion, but he or she could not compel the mother to comply. Finally, during the third trimester, the time when substance abuse is most harmful to fetuses, the state may be able to intervene on the fetus' behalf.[116]

Under *Roe, Jefferson*, and *Taft*, fetal rights attach at viability, and at that point the state can intrude on a mother's constitutionally protected rights to preserve the life and health of the child. The first step would be for the physician to report the alleged child abuse to the appropriate state agecy.[117] The state agency would investigate the matter and prescribe counseling if necessary. If these methods do not stop the abuse, then and only then will the state step in to protect the fetus. The state agency would then petition the court under Section 300 to have the fetus adjudged a dependent minor.[118] Once the court obtained jurisdiction over the fetus, it could then compel the mother to undergo whatever treatment thought necessary to protect the fetus.[119] The court could award the state agency custody to authorize any necessary treatment. The state agency would have custody of the fetus until its birth, or until custody could safely be returned to the mother.[120]

This solution to the problem is desirable for many reasons. A legislative mandate would eliminate judicial confusion. Judges would know the circumstances under which they could protect a fetus from maternal abuse. An amendment to the neglect and dependency statutes is preferable to an extension of the penal codes because the state's main purpose should be to protect the fetus, not punish the addicted mother.[121] Also, precedent supports the extension of neglect and dependency statutes to protect the unborn.[122] Finally, the procedural safeguards that accompany these statutes would protect the mother's right to privacy until the fetus' right to a healthy birth becomes paramount.[123]

B. Alternative Solution

In the absence of legislative action, courts could protect a viable fetus from maternal abuse by interpreting the present neglect and dependency statutes in favor of the unborn child.[124] However, this has not occurred in some jurisdictions. For example, a California court refused to interpret the neglect and dependency statutes to include protections for the fetus.[125] The court said that extending the statute to include a fetus is the task of the legislature.[126] Thus, in states like California, revised legislation appears to be the only way to protect the unborn. However, other jurisdictions are free to make such an interpretation in the absence of a contrary holding. Precedent exists for this interpretation and, if applied within the constraints of *Roe*, it would be constitutional.[127] When legislators fail to act, the courts should assume the role of decision maker, reflecting in their decisions the mandates of society.[128] The case presented in this chapter's introduction could have been resolved the same way without legislative amendment if the court had interpreted the state neglect and dependency statutes to include the fetus, and applied the statutes within the constitutional boundaries of *Roe*.

Ultimately, the United States Supreme Court has the last word in resolving the conflict of rights between a mother and a fetus. The justices' ideologies undoubtedly affect their decisions on controversial issues. The next section examines the practicability of this proposal in relation to the changing ideological makeup of the Supreme Court.

V. A LOOK INTO THE FUTURE

The highly controversial issue of women's rights during pregnancy, especially as it pertains to abortion, will unquestionably be affected by new appointments to the Supreme Court. The Court's opinion about a mother's right to privacy may be undergoing a reformation. Predicting the future status of a woman's right to privacy is at best an educated guess. Nonetheless, a discussion of the present and possible future ideological composition of the Court is necessary to give credence to the proposal offered in Section IV. This proposal invites criticism because it attempts to resolve a highly emotional and controversial issue. Some complain that it infringes too greatly on the mother's right to privacy. Others suggest that it does not sufficiently protect the fetus from maternal abuses. These criticisms reflect the traditional polar views of conservatives and liberals on the subject of human rights.

The United States Supreme Court, as the highest court in the nation, is more and more frequently called upon to make social judgments. The determination of whether or not a proposal allowing for state-enforced incarceration of a woman for the protection of her unborn child is constitutional may depend on which particular men and women are selected to fill the upcoming vacancies on the Court.

Presently, the liberal view of abortion and fetal rights is also the majority view of the Court. However, the conservative faction is gaining power with each new Reagan appointee. This raises many questions about the decisions a conservative court may reach on such controversial issues as abortion and fetal rights. In attempting to answer these questions, one must begin by examining the views of each of the justices comprising the Court. A recently decided Supreme Court case provides a vehicle for such assessment.

Thornburgh v. American College of Obstetricians and Gynecologists was decided on June 11, 1986.[129] On the face of it, it appears to be just another case of a state attempting to regulate abortion procedures. Thus, it is very reminiscent of *Akron v. Akron Center for Reproductive Health, Inc.*[130] and *Planned Parenthood Assn. of Kansas City, Mo., Inc. v. Ashcroft.*[131] Again, the Court held the legislation unconstitutional.

It is not the holding of the case, however, that is interesting. Rather, it is the increasing disparity between Court conservatives and liberals, which provides insight into the future.

Justice Blackmun authored the recent *Thornburgh* opinion, just as he authored the 1973 *Roe* opinion. Blackmun is 77-years-old and still a staunch supporter of the *Roe* framework. He is reportedly unwilling to resign if his successor would be likely to overturn the abortion ruling.[132] In *Thornburgh*, Blackmun defends his position in this way:

> Constitutional rights do not have easily ascertainable boundaries, and controversy over the meaning of our Nation's most majestic guarantees frequently has been turbulent. As judges, however, we are sworn to uphold the law even when its content gives rise to bitter dispute. [citations omitted] We recognized at the very beginning of our opinion in *Roe*, 410 U.S. at 116, that abortion raises moral and spiritual questions over which honorable persons can disagree sincerely and profoundly. But those disagreements did not then and do not now relieve us of our duty to apply the Constitution faithfully.
>
> Our cases long have recognized that the Constitution embodies a promise tht a certain private sphere of individual liberty will be kept largely beyond the reach of government. [citations omitted] That promise extends to women as well as men. Few decisions are more personal and intimate, more properly private, or more basic to individual dignity and autonomy than a woman's decision—with the guidance of her physician and within the limits specified in *Roe*—whether to end her pregnancy. A woman's right to make that choice freely is fundamental. Any other result, in our view, would protect inadequately a central part of the sphere of liberty that our law guarantees equally to all.[133]

This unequivocal reaffirmation of the principles underlying *Roe* was joined by Justices Brennan, Marshall, Powell and Stevens. It represents the liberal position—the position that prevents a state from infringing too deeply on a pregnant woman's right to privacy. Since our proposal fits within the *Roe* framework, it is likely to be viewed favorably by this majority. However, this position is espoused by only 5 justices. This slim majority may be slipping, given the possibility of additional conservative appointees.

Justice White wrote a powerful dissent in *Thornburugh*. He states: "In my view, the time has come to recognize that *Roe v. Wade* . . . departs from a proper understanding of the Constitution, and to overrule it."[134] White continues, at length, to reexamine the basic foundations of the *Roe* opinion, and concludes that the Constitution does not protect a woman's right to have an abortion. He contends that the right to an abortion is too different from the other rights protected under the rubric of personal or family privacy and autonomy, and that the trimester framework enunciated in *Roe* is at best arbitary since it fails to protect the lives of nonviable fetuses. He argues that, once the trimester framework of *Roe* is rejected, restrictions and even outright prohibitions on abortions would become a state's prerogative.[135]

Justice White is joined in his opinion by Justice Rehnquist. Justices Burger and O'Connor, in separate dissenting opinions, also claim that it is time to reexamine *Roe v. Wade*. An opinion by this conservative faction would most likely deny that abortion is a constitutional issue at all, thus making it a matter for each state to resolve. This would enable a state to regulate abortions, or even abolish them altogether.

Our proposal could well straddle the fine line between the conservative and liberal viewpoints on abortion and fetal rights. It would appeal to the liberals because of its confinement within the *Roe* framework. It would also appeal to the conservatives because of its emphasis on fetal rights. Indeed, the conservative faction might be tempted to extend its protection of fetal rights beyond what these authors advocate and intervene earlier in a woman's pregnancy.

Since the present status of the law was achieved by a 5–4 vote, a conservative majority opinion may become a reality in the near future. Each new Reagan appointment brings this possibility closer. Although the recent replacement of Chief Justice Burger with William Rehnquist just replaces one conservative with another, some commentators feel that Rehnquist will do much to push the Court considerably to the right.[136]

As an Associate Justice, Rehnquist was a consistent defender of states' rights against federal intrusion. He has also consistently resisted the efforts of other Justices to protect individual rights through their broader interpretation of the Constitution. He is a staunch opponent of the exclusionary rule, a consistent proponent of the death penalty, and one of the dissenters in *Roe v. Wade*.[137] As Chief Justice, his opinion-assigning power is expected to enable him to set the terms of the debate and forge majorities that espouse his positions.[138]

The appointment of Antonin Scalia to the Court will further aid Rehnquists's crusade. Scalia, a father of nine, has a "deeply developed philosophy based on the principles of strict separation of powers and disdain for far-reaching federal remedies for social problems."[139] Many believe that Scalia will vote as a classic conservative, to let states decide the abortion issue, to limit affirmative action plans, to limit the rights of criminal defendants, and to narrowly interpret the First Amendment rights of the press.[140] These recent changes on the Court are unlikely to produce any drastic changes in the Court's decisions in the immediate future. However, the possibility of additional appointments of conservative Justices may have a profound effect on the Court's decisions. The future may very well bring many drastic changes, such as curtailing the rights of pregnant women to make basic decisions about their pregnancies. The balance of rights between a mother and a fetus is a delicate one. This article offers one solution for resolving the inherent conflict.

CONCLUSION

The fetus has a right to be born healthy. The state may intervene to assure the fetus' well-being under statute and case law. Once a woman decides to carry the pregnancy to term, she is obligated to care for her unborn child. If she fails to take proper care of herself, and the fetus is in danger, the state may interfere and declare the fetus to be neglected or abused, and appoint a guardian to authorize the necessary treatment. State intervention is warranted when the fetus' life and health is threatened as a result of maternal substance abuse. A state should compel women to be free of drug and alcohol addiction until the child is born or the pregnancy is terminated. Presently, mothers have a choice. They can commit themselves to doing everything possible to insure the healthy birth of their baby, or they can terminate their pregnancy within the first few months. However, the future legal environment may not offer them the luxury of such a choice.

REFERENCES

1. *N.Y. Times*, Apr. 27, 1983 at 1, col. 4. This case is included as an example of cases in which a conflict arose between the rights of a mother and the rights of her unborn child. *See also* Andrews, *A Delicate Condition*, **Student Law**, May 1985, at 30. This author questions whether or not the law should police pregnancies in order to protect the fetus' well-being.

2. "Compelling state interest" is a term used in modern equal-protection or due-process cases. The requirement that the state have a compelling interest in furthering its goal indicates that the Court is giving the regulation a high standard of review commonly called "strict scrutiny." The Court uses this standard of review when a state action infringes on a right the Court deems to be fundamental or on a class of persons the Court has decided is suspect. *See generally* ***J. Nowak, R. Rotunda & J. Young, Constitutional Law*** 418–19 (2d ed. 1983).

3. Roe v. Wade, 410 U.S. 113 (1973). *See also infra* notes 45–55 and accompanying text.

4. *Id.*

5. ***J. Pritchard & P. MacDonald, Williams Obstetrics*** 329 (16th ed. 1980).

6. *Id.* at 205. The maternal diet is the source of nutrients supplied to the fetus. Much of what a mother eats, drinks, or ingests penetrates the placenta and reaches the fetus. *Id.*

7. ***Pritchard & MacDonald***, *supra* note 5, at 329.

8. *Id.*

9. Lenow, *The Fetus as a Patient: Emerging Rights as a Person?*, 9 ***Am. J. of L. & Med.*** 1, 15 (1983). The author believes that, more and more frequently, the fetus will have a separate physician and be treated separately from its mother.

10. *See* Manning, Lange, Morrison & Harman, *Treatment of the Fetus in Utero: Evolving Concepts*, 27 ***Clinical Obstet. & Gynecol.*** 378 (1984).

11. One of the rarer techniques that may raise conflicts between the rights of a mother and her fetus is fetal surgery. The ability to view and evaluate the fetus while still in the

mother's womb now allows physicians to diagnose fetal diseases or malformations. Physicians may treat some of these conditions by fetal surgery. *Id.* at 387. The use of these procedures is currently very rare, and physicians reserve treatment for a few specific disorders. *Id.* at 388.

12. *See infra* notes 16 & 19.

13. This chapter uses the term "substance abuser" to describe a person who abuses or is addicted to drugs or alcohol.

14. *See infra* notes 16 & 19.

15. *See* Acker, Sachs, Tracey & Wise, *Abruptio Placentae Associated with Cocaine Use*, 146 ***Am J. Obstet. Gynecol.*** 220 (1983). Medical complications of cocaine use include hypertension, seizures, respiratory arrest, and cardiac failure. Cocaine use by a pregnant woman can cause the placenta to separate from the site of implantation before delivery of the fetus, causing the infant to be stillborn or developmentally impaired. *Id.* at 220–21.

16. *See* Hutchings, *Methadone and Heroin During Pregnancy: A Review of Behavioral Effects in Human and Animal Offspring*, 4 ***Neurobehavioral Toxicology & Teratology*** 429 (1982). Studies show that prenatal exposure to heroin or methadone produces effects that occur in two stages. Hyperactivity and disturbed sleep characterize the early phase, lasting from 12 weeks to 6 months. These symptoms result from the slow clearance of the drug from the neonatal tissues. Impaired organizational and perceptual abilities, poor self-adjustment and hyperactivity characterize the second phase, which is even seen in preschool-aged children. *Id.* The author points out that in approximately 3 to 5 births, infants are passively addicted to heroin or methadone. Thus, the birth rate of the addicted population is about 3,000 per year in New York City alone. *Id.*

17. *See, e.g., Feeding America's Habit: A Booming Demand Frustrates Law-Enforcement Effort*, ***Newsweek***, Feb. 27, 1985, at 22–23 (increasing demand for cocaine).

18. Jones, Smith, Streissguth & Myrianthopoulos, *Outcome in Offspring of Chronic Alcoholic Women*, 1974 ***The Lancet*** 1076–78. The author states that the frequency of adverse outcome in the pregnancies of chronically alcoholic women is great; therefore, women should seriously consider early termination of the pregnancy. *Id.* at 1076.

19. *See* Nace, *Peidemiology of Alcoholism and Prospects for Treatment*, 35 ***Ann. Rev. Med.*** 293 (1984). The author suggests that the 1970s was a decade of increase in alcohol consumption for millions of Americans. "Alcoholic beverages became more accessible in more states, the drinking age was lowered, the number of outlets increased, and the price of alcohol rose less, relative to other consumer products." *Id.* at 294.

20. Kruse, *Alcohol Use in Pregnancy*, 29 ***Am. Fam. Prac.*** 199 (1984). Aristotle noticed that drunken women often gave birth to abnormal infants. In the 1700s, Liverpool physicians reported a high rate of stillbirths and early deaths among the offspring of alcoholic mothers. They noticed however, that if alcoholic women abstained from alcohol during subsequent pregnancies, the offspring were likely to be normal. *Id.* at 199.

21. Lemoine, Haronssedu & Boroteryer, *Les Enfants de Parents Alcooliqueus: Anomalies Observees a Propos de 127 Cas*, 25 ***Ouest Med.*** 476 (1968).

22. Jones & Smith, *Recognition of the Fetal Alcohol Syndrome in Early Infancy*, 2 ***The Lancet*** 999 (1973).

23. Rosett, *Patterns of Alcohol Consumption and Fetal Development*, 61 ***Obstet. & Gynecol.*** 539 (1983). Medical experts associate fetal alcohol syndrome with a heavy intake of alcohol during pregnancy. "Heavy intake" means 45 drinks per month or more

than five on any single occasion. *Id.* "Moderate intake" means more than one drink per month, but never more than five drinks on any single occasion. *Id.*

24. Kruse, *supra* note 20, at 201. Infants with fetal alcohol syndrome suffer from three specific types of abnormalities. These include: 1) Craniofacial abnormalities, such as microcephaly, short upturned nose, thin upper lip, cleft lip and palate; 2) Developmental abnormalities, such as prenatal growth retardation and postnatal growth deficiency; and 3) Neurologic abnormalities, such as mental retardation, learning disabilities, behavioral disorders, sleep and speed disorders, and poor sucking reflex. *Id.*

About one in 750 children born in the United States will have symptoms of fetal alcohol syndrome. Infants of women who have consumed three-to-five drinks per day have a 10 to 30 percent chance of suffering from fetal alcohol syndrome. The risk of growth, neurological, or genetic abnormalities is 50 to 70 percent for these infants. *Id.*

The frequency of all abnormalities in infants born to alcoholic mothers is twice as great as the frequency of abnormalities in infants of women who consumed little or no alcohol during pregnancy. *See* Oullette, *Adverse Effects on Offspring of Maternal Alcohol Abuse During Pregnancy*, 297 ***New Eng. J. of Med.*** 528 (1977). When viewed in conjunction with the increasing incidence of alcohol use in young women, these statistics are alarming. *See* Nace, *supra* note 19, at 295. This study states that alcohol use is on the rise in the U.S. Alcoholism has increased five to nine percent in women from 1967 to 1970. *Id.*

25. *See* Kruse, *supra* note 24, at 201. Many of these abnormalities are permanent. *Id.*

26. *Id. See also* Rosette, *supra* note 23, at 544–45. The site of greatest damage from alcohol is the human central nervous system, which controls the growth and development of the brain and spinal chord. The central nervous system undergoes rapid growth during the third trimester. Thus, reducing alcohol intake use during that time can increase the chances that the fetus will be normal. *Id.*

27. *Roe v. Wade*, 410 U.S. 113 (1973). *See also* Coleman, *Roe v. Wade: A Retrospective Look at a Judicial Oxymoron*, 29 ***St. Louis U.L.J.*** 7, 13–14 (1984).

28. *See infra* notes 91–109 and accompanying test. *See also Women's Rights vs. Fetal Rights Looms as Thorny and Divisive Issue*, The Wall St. J., Apr. 12, 1985, at 1, col. 4. The article states:

> At the other extreme is a growing number of people who contend that the state's interest in protecting a fetus against maternal negligence is just as strong as its interest in protecting a child against parental child abuse. Unlike right-to-life groups that advance fetal rights as part of an argument against abortion, these people generally support the woman's right to abortion, but insist that once she decides to carry the fetus to term, she loses some of her constitutionally protected bodily freedom and is obliged to do all she reasonably can to insure the birth of a healthy baby." *Id.*

29. *See* ***Blackstone, Commentaries*** *130. "An infant *en ventre sa mere* [in the mother's womb] is supposed in law to be born for many purposes. It is capable of having a legacy, or surrender of a copyhold estate, made to it. It may have a guardian assigned to it; and it is enabled to have an estate limited to its use, and to take afterwards by such limitation, as if it were then actually born."

30. *See generally* Shaw & Damme, *Legal Status of the Fetus*, in ***Genetics and the Law I*** (1976).

31. *Id.*

32. 2 Cal. 3d 619, 470 P.2d 617, 87 Cal. Rptr. 481 (1970) (violent attack on mother late in pregnancy found to be the cause of stillbirth).

33. *Id.* at 631, 470 P.2d at 615, 87 Cal. Rpr. at 488. *See also* King, *The Juridical Status of the Fetus: A Proposal for Legal Protection of the Unborn*, 77 ***Mich. L. Rev.*** 1647, 1662–63 (1979).

34. ***Cal. Penal Code*** § 187 (West 1970 & Supp. 1985).

35. ***Cal. Penal Code*** § 270 (West 1970 & Supp. 1985).

36. *Id.* The statute states: "A child conceived but not yet born is deemed an existing person insofar as this section is concerned." *Id.*

37. *See In re* Baby X, No. 77–1557 (6th Jud. Cir. Oakland City, Mich.). *But see* Reyes v. Superior Court, 75 Cal. App. 3d 214, 141 Cal. Rptr. 912 (1977) (court refused to indict drug-addicted mother under ***Cal. Penal Code*** § 273(a), the felony child endangerment statute).

38. *See*, Levine, *The Right of the Fetus to Be Born Free of Drug Addiction*, 7 ***U.C. Davis L. Rev.*** 45, 48 (1974).

39. *See* Bonbrest v. Kotz, 65 F. Supp. 138 (D.D.C. 1946).

40. *See, e.g.*, Hornbuckle v. Plantation Pipe Line, 212 Ga. 504, 93 S.E.2d 727 (1956). *See also* King, *supra* note 33, at 1660–64.

41. *See* Justus v. Atchison, 19 Cal. 3d 564, 565 P.2d 122, 139 Cal. Rptr. 97 (1977).

42. *See* Verkennes v. Corniea, 299 Minn. 365, 38 N.W.2d 838 (1949).

43. *See infra* text accompanying notes 48–55.

44. *Id.*

45. 410 U.S. 113 (1973).

46. 381 U.S. 479 (1965). In *Griswold v. Connecticut*, petitioners challenged the constitutionality of two Connecticut statutes that prohibited the practice of contraception and the providing of information about contraception. The Supreme Court held the statutes unconstitutional because they violated the fundamental right to marital privacy (found in the "penumbra" of the Bill of Rights) and no compelling interest was involved. *Id. See also* King, *supra* note 33, at 1665 (recognition of rights relating to childbearing was initiated in *Griswold*).

47. *See, e.g.*, Eisenstadt v. Baird, 405 U.S. 438 (1972). In *Eisenstadt* the petitioner challenged the constitutionality of a statute prohibiting the dispensing of contraceptives to unmarried persons. The Supreme Court held the statute unconstitutional as a denial of equal protection. *Id.* at 446–47. In addition, the Court noted, "if the right to privacy means anything, it is the right of the individual, married or single, to be free from unwarranted governmental intrusion into matters so fundamentally affecting a person as the decision whether to bear or beget a child." *Id.* at 453.

48. 410 U.S. 113 (1973).

49. *Id.* at 165.

50. *Id.* at 165–66. *See also* King, *supra* note 33, at 1650. The author emphasizes that the woman's right to privacy is qualified. *Id.*

51. 410 U.S. at 162–64. The Court held that the state had two possible important interests, either of which could become more compelling at different times during pregnancy. The state could assert an interest in maternal health and in potential life. *Id. See also* Coleman, *supra* note 27, at 13.

52. 410 U.S. at 164–65. The state's interest in maternal health is not compelling during the first trimester (approximately the first twelve weeks) of pregnancy because the risks associated with childbirth are greater than the risks of early abortion. Nor is the state's interest in protecting potential life compelling at this time, because the fetus is not yet viable. *Id.*

See Coleman, *supra* note 27, at 13–14. The author criticizes the *Roe* decision for its logical inconsistency. *Id.* at 11–12. *But see* King, supra note 33, at 1647–57 (the *Roe* decision is conceptually sound in its reliance on viability as the point at which fetal rights attach).

53. 410 U.S. at 164–65. The state's interest in maternal health becomes compelling during the second trimester when the risk of maternal death from abortion is greater than or equal to the risk of death from childbirth. The state may regulate abortions at this point. *Id. See also* articles cited *supra* note 52.

54. 410 U.S. at 164–65. In the third trimester of pregnancy, the fetus becomes potentially viable and the state's interest in protecting potential life becomes compelling. *Id. See also* articles cited *supra* note 52.

55. 410 U.S. at 160.

56. ***Pritchard & MacDonald*** *supra* note 5, at 587.

57. Lenow, *supra* note 9, at 11. Physicians consider fetal age and weight, and the stage of development of the major organ systems, in assessing viability. *Id.*

58. 410 U.S. at 159. The Court held that the moment a fetus became potentially viable, the interest in potential life became compelling. At this point, the state could prohibit abortion. *Id.*

59. Planned Parenthood of Central Missouri v. Danforth, 428 U.S. 52 (1976). *See also* Lenow, *supra* note 9, at 11 (analysis of each issue of viability on a case-by-case basis, reiterates the medical profession's role in deciding viability).

60. 428 U.S. 52 (1976).

61. ***Mo. Ann. Stat.*** § 188.015(3) (Vernon Supp. 1975).

62. 428 U.S. at 63. *See also* Lenow, *supra* note 9, at 12.

63. 439 U.S. 379 (1979). In *Coalutti v. Franklin*, the plaintiff challenged a Pennsylvania abortion statute that attempted to limit the physician's broad discretion in determining viability. The Court held the statute invalid for vagueness, and repeated that the determination of viability is to be made by physicians and not by legislators. *Id.* at 387–89.

64. *Id.* at 400. *See also* Lenow, *supra* note 9, at 11.

65. 103 S. Ct. 2581 (1983).

66. Viability is a point in time that is not readily discernible and varies from fetus to fetus. The *Roe* framework was based on two notions. As long as abortions are safer than childbirth, the woman's privacy right overrides the fetus' right to life. Once the fetus becomes viable and abortions are no longer safer than childbirth, the fetus' right to life becomes superior to the woman's privacy right. Advances in medicine may one day be responsible for viability and safe abortions being possible at the same moment in pregnancy, thereby commingling two notions that the Supreme Court had assumed were distinct events for purposes of their analysis in *Roe*.

67. 103 S. Ct. at 2495. Justice O'Connor's dissenting opinion predicts the future demise of the trimester approach. She suggests that the *Roe* framework will become more and more unworkable as the viability line is obscured by medical advances. *Id.* at 2507 (O'Connor, J., dissenting). *See also* Coleman, *supra* note 27, at 15.

68. *See generally* King, *supra* note 33.

69. King, *supra* note 33, at 1676.

70. Manning, Lange, Morrison, & Harman, *supra* note 10, at 378–79 (perinatal mortality has declined due to recent medical breakthroughs in diagnosis and treatment of pereinatal difficulties).

71. King, *supra* note 33, at 1667 (when the fetus becomes capable of a separate existence, it should be granted the benefit of the doubt regarding its ability to contribute to society).

72. *Id.* at 1679–87 (some of the difficulties surrounding the viability standard are: complexity of the determination, the Supreme Court's extraordinary deference to the medical profession on the subject, the problem of applying the viability standard in situations other than abortion, the fact that viability can shift with advances in medical technology, and the fact that viability represents a moment in fetal development that is not readily apparent to lay persons or physicians).

73. *Id.* at 1682 (author suggests the assertion of a presumption of viability at 25 weeks, the earliest point at which fetal survival has been documented). *Id.* at 1679 & n.145. The author mentions possible ways in which the presumption may be rebutted. *Id.* at 1682.

74. *See, e.g.*, Superintendent of Belchertown State School v. Saikewicz, 373 Mass. 728, 370 N.E.2d 417 (1977). *See also In re* Quinlan, 70 N.J. 10, 355 A.2d 647 (1976).

75. *See, e.g.*, Scholendorff v. Society of New York Hospital, 211 N.Y. 125, 129, 105 N.E. 92, 93 (1914).

76. *See, e.g., In re* Melideo, 88 Misc.2d 974, 390 N.E.2d 523 (N.Y. Sup. Ct. 1976).

77. Jacobsen v. Massachusetts, 197 U.S. 11 (1904). *See also* Finamore, *Jefferson v. Griffin Spaulding County Hospital Authority: Court Ordered Surgery to Protect the Life of an Unborn Child*, 9 ***Am. J. of L. & Med.*** 83, 91 (1983).

78. *In re* President and Directors of Georgetown College, Inc., 331 F.2d 1000 (D.C. Cir. 1964), involved a woman who refused to have a blood transfusion because of her religious beliefs. The court ordered her to undergo treatment. The court noted that the patient had a seven-month-old dependent child. *Id.* at 1008. The court also relied on the following factors:

1. The patient did not want to die;
2. The situation was life-threatening;
3. The patient was too weak to make a rational decision on her own behalf.
   Id. at 1008–09.

79. *Id.*

80. Jacobsen v. Massachusetts, 197 U.S. 11 (1904) (the court ordered the individual to have a smallpox vaccination because refusal of treatment would endanger others).

81. *See supra* notes 68–73 and accompanying text.

82. 412 N.J. 421, 201 A.2d 537, *cert. denied*, 377 U.S. 985 (1974).

83. *Id.* at 422, 201 A.2d at 538.

84. *See supra* note 54.

85. *See supra* note 80.

86. 247 Ga. 86, 274 S.E.2d 457 (1981).

87. *Id.* at 86, 274 S.E.2d at 457.

88. *Id.*

89. *Id.* at 87, 274 S.E.2d at 458 (construing ***Ga. Code Ann.*** § 26–1202 (1973)).

90. *Id.* at 87, 274 S.E.2d at 459.

91. ***Ga. Code Ann.*** § 24A–401(h)(i) (1973).

92. *Jefferson*, 247 Ga. at 88, 274 S.E.2d at 459.

93. 247 Ga. at 90, 274 S.E.2d at 460 (Hill, J., concurring). Justice Hill's concurrence noted, "We weighed the right of the mother to practice her religion and to refuse surgery on herself against her unborn child's right to live. We found in favor of the child's right to live." *Id.*

94. Lenow, *supra* note 9, at 22, The author states: "while the prohibition of abortion considered in *Roe* placed the state in the position of passively restricting the choices available to the pregnant woman, *Jefferson* authorizes active state participation in facilitating the birth of a viable fetus." *Id.*

95. Finamore, *Jefferson v. Griffin Spalding County Hospital Authority: Court-Ordered Surgery to Protect the Life of an Unborn Child*, 9 ***Am. J. of L. & Med.*** 83, 88 (1983). The author also suggests that *Jefferson* raises the possibility of intrusive state restrictions on the mother's conduct, such as prohibiting smoking or drinking, without proof of detriment to the unborn child. *Id.* at 88 n. 35.

96. *Id.* at 92.

97. 388 Mass. 381, 446 N.E.2d 395 (1983).

98. *Id.* at 332 n.2, 446 N.E.2d at 396 n.2.

99. *Id.* at 334 n.4, 446 N.E.2d at 397 n.4.

100. *Id.* at 334, 446 N.E.2d at 397.

101. *See supra* notes 86–99 and accompanying text.

102. *See supra* note 99 and accompanying text.

103. Finamore, *supra* note 95, at 101.

104. *Id.*

105. *See supra* note 54 and accompanying text.

106. *See supra* text accompanying notes 48–58 and 86–93.

107. *See* Ament, *The Right to be Well Born*, ***J. Leg. Med.***, Nov.-Dec. 1974, at 24.

108. *See* Capron, *The Continuing Wrong of Wrongful Life*, ***Genetics & the Law II***, 1980, at 91. *See also* Turpin v. Sortini, 119 Cal. App. 3d 690, 696, 174 Cal. Rptr. 128, 132 (1981).

109. *See, e.g., supra* notes 33–36 and accompanying text.

110. ***Cal. Welf. & Inst. Code*** § 300 (West 1972 & Supp. 1985). Section 300 states: any person under the age of 18 years who comes within any of the following descriptions is within the jurisdiction of the juvenile court, which may adjudge such person to be a dependent child of the court:

(a) who is in need of proper and effective parental care or control and has no parent or guardian willing to exercise or capable of exercising proper and effective parental care or control solely because of a physical disability, including, but not limited to, a defect in visual or auditory functions of his or her body, unless the court finds that the disability prevents the parent from exercising such care or control.

(b) who is destitute, or who is not provided with the necessities of life, or who is not provided with a home or suitable place of abode.

(c) who is physically dangerous to the public because of a mental or physical deficiency, disorder, or abnormality.

(d) whose home is an unfit place for him by reason of neglect, cruelty, depravity, or physical abuse of either of his parents, or of his guardian or other person in whose custody or care he is.

(e) who has been freed for adoption from one or both parents for 12 months by either relinquishment or termination of parental rights and for whom an interlocutory decree has not been granted pursuant to Section 224n of the Civil Code or an adoption petition has not been granted.

111. *Id.*

112. *See, e.g.*, Matter of LaShonda B., 95 Cal. App. 3d 593, 157 Cal. Rptr. 280 (1979).

113. Due Process requires the state to appoint counsel for indigent parents in child dependency proceedings, Cleaver v. Wilcox, 499 F.2d 940 (9th Cir. 1974), to provide proper notice and opportunity to be heard, *In re* Jeremy S.C., 109 Cal. App. 3d 384, 167 Cal. Rptr. 283 (1980), and to use a "clear and convincing" evidence standard to support the conclusion that a child is dependent, *In re* Jamie M. 134 Cal. App. 3d 530, 184 Cal. Rptr. 778 (1982).

Cal. Welf. & Inst. Code § 319 (West 1972 & Supp. 1985) (requires state to make use of referral methods that would facilitate return of child home and report on availability of such services to court).

114. *See supra* note 52 and accompanying text.

115. *See supra* note 53 and accompanying text.

116. *See supra* note 26.

117. It is the responsibility of physicians as well as teachers, day-care operators, and others to report suspected child abuse to the proper state authority. ***Cal. Penal Code*** §§ 11165–11166 (West 1972 & Supp. 1985). For a discussion and listing of these statutes, *see* ***J. Costa & G. Nelson, Child Abuse and Neglect: Legislation, Reporting and Prevention*** (1978). *See also* Paulsen, *Child Abuse Reporting Laws: The Shape of Legislation*, 67 ***Colum. L. Rev.*** 1 (1967). If a fetus is analogous to a dependent child, then fetal abuse should be reported as well. *See supra* notes 69–71 and accompanying text.

118. This was the approach used in Jefferson. *See supra* notes 90–91 and accompanying text.

119. The court must carefully analyze the treatment ordered and balance the chance of benefit to the fetus against risk of harm to the mother. In *Jefferson*, the chance for success well outweighed the risk. *See supra* notes 93 and accompanying text. But if this is not the case, courts should be more reluctant to order treatment.

120. *See supra* note 90 and accompanying text.

121. *See supra* note 112 and accompanying text.

122. *See supra* note 90 and accompanying text.

123. Although the authors of this chapter feel that states neglect and dependency statutues are the most susceptible to the proposed reform, other statutes could be interpreted to protect fetuses from substance abuse as well. State civil commitment statutes are possible vehicles for fetal protection. *See* Levine *supra* note 38, at 54.

For example, California Welfare and Institutions Code, Section 3000 was designed to protect addicts, potential addicts, and society-at-large from narcotics addiction. *See* ***Cal. Welf. & Inst. Code*** §3000 (West 1972 & Supp. 1985).

The state, under the doctrine of *parens patriae*, can compel the treatment of addicts for these purposes. Section 3000 provides in part:

> It is the intent of the legislature that persons addicted to narcotics, or who by reason of repeated uses of narcotics are in imminent danger of becoming addicted, shall be treated for such condition and its underlying causes, and that such treatment shall be carried out for nonpunitive purposes, not only for the protection of the addict or persons in imminent danger of addiction, but also for the prevention of the contamination of others and the protection of the public.

Courts have held that the purposes of Section 3000 is not only to protect the addict, but to prevent the contamination of others as well. *See, e.g.*, People v. Navarro, 7 Cal.

App. 3d 248, 497 P.2d 481, 102 Cal. Rptr. 137 (1952). A fetus could be considered an "other" within the meaning of the statute.

State civil commitment statutes may provide for the treatment of alcoholics as well. For example, California Welfare and Institutions Code, Section 5225 provides for involuntary treatment of a criminal defendant who, as a result of chronic alcoholism, is a danger to herself or to others. *See* ***Cal. Welf. & Inst. Code.*** § 5225 (West 1972 & Supp. 1985). The argument that a fetus is an "other" within the meaning of the statute could be used here as well to extend protection to fetuses of alcoholic women.

Even though state civil commitment statutes do not specifically protect fetuses, a favorable interpretation could lead to that result.

124. Legislative action is often slow when the proposed legislation has moral overtones. Justice Blackmun recognized this fact in the opening paragraphs of the *Roe* decision and states, "our task, of course, is to resolve the issue by constitutional measurement, free of emotion and of predilection." Roe v. Wade, 410 U.S. 113, 116 (1973).

125. Matter of Steven G.S., 126 Cal. App. 3d 23, 25, 178 Cal. Rptr 525, 526 (1981).

126. *Id.*

127. *See supra* note 90 and accompanying text.

128. *Roe v. Wade*, 410 U.S. 113 (1973). The *Roe* decision is an example of one situation where the Court had to act when legislators failed to remove archaic laws from the books. The decision virtually overruled legislation in all 50 states. The Texas statutes held unconstitutional by the Court ". . . are typical of those that have been in effect in many states for approximately a century." *Id.* at 116.

129. 54 U.S.L.W. 4618 (U.S. June 10, 1986).

130. 103 S. Ct. 2581 (1983).

131. 462 U.S. 476 (1983).

132. *Reagan Justice*, ***Newsweek***, June 30, 1986, at 15.

133. 54 U.S.L.W. at 4625.

134. *Id.* at 4629.

135. *Id.* at 4631.

136. *Reagan's Mr. Right*, ***Time***, June 30, 1986, at 24–25.

137. *Id.* at 27.

138. *Id.* at 29.

139. *Id.* at 29.

140. *Reagan Justice*, ***Newsweek***, June 30, 1986, at 18–19; *Reagan's Mr. Right*, ***Time***, June 30, 1986, at 30–33.

10. Euthanasia: Where Are We? Where Are We Going?

Marvin S. Fish, Esquire

For the past decade, on the subject of euthanasia the courts of New Jersey have been wrestling with the Angel of Death, trying to determine when his will is irresistible and when, although it might be resisted, it ought not to be. Steeped in moral convictions as to the sanctity of life and the inappropriateness of the interference of man in the apparent workings of God, we have been lately forced to interface with technological developments whose potential applications often give us the power to choose exactly when the moment of death will occur. Our values of self-determination and individual freedom pull us in one direction here; our value of equal justice for all pulls us in an opposite one. Moreover, the entire conflict is intertwined with a sense of paternalism which, imbued by our theologically nourished conscience, influences us to seek and to follow some universally acceptable standard of right.

Now that issues like cost-effectiveness, PROs, third-party payers, taxation, limited staff and allocation of resources are achieving priority, we find ourselves with a new focus. Having barely adjusted to "bio-ethics," we now must move into the realm of "econo-ethics."

New Jersey has dealt with two types of terminally ill patients. One is the competent patient. Competence has been defined as having " . . . sufficient mind to reasonably understand the condition, the nature, and effect of the proposed treatment, and the attendant risks in pursuing the treatment and not pursuing the treatment." *In re Schiller*, 148 NJ Super at 180–181, 372 A.2d at 367 (1977).

The saga really begins with *Schloendorff v. Society of New York Hosp.*, 211 NY 125, 129–130, 105 N.E. 92, 93 (1914), as recognized in *In re Quinlan*, 70

NJ 10, 335 A.2d 647 (1976), and repeated in *The Matter of Conroy*, 98 NJ 321 at 346 (1985), in the words "a competent adult person generally has the right to decline to have any medical treatment initiated or continued." The Court rests this conclusion on the Common-Law right to self-determination and the right to privacy found in both the New Jersey and the United States Constitutions. Such a right is not without qualification, and the Court deals with the state's interests, which must also be considered.

The second type of patient is the one who is incompetent at the time a decision needs to be made. Such a patient might have made known his desires before becoming incompetent or might not have. If they were made known before, then they will be followed. *Conroy* deals with the quest for such a determination and the course to be followed if it cannot be determined.

Claire Conroy was an eighty-four-year-old nursing home resident who suffered from serious and irreversible physical and mental impairments, including arteriosclerotic heart disease, hypertension, and diabetes. Her condition eventually reached a point where she could not speak or swallow sufficient amounts of nutrients and water to sustain herself. She was fed and medicated through a nasogastric tube. She was not in control of her excretory functions. Miss Conroy could move to a minor extent, and she occasionally smiled or moaned in response to certain stimuli.

Thomas C. Whittemore, Claire Conroy's nephew and guardian, sought court permission to remove his incompetent aunt's nasogastric tube. The application was opposed by Miss Conroy's guardian *ad litem*.

At trial, the evidence indicated that Claire Conroy was unable to move from a semifetal position, that her intellectual capacity was very limited, and that her mental condition would probably never improve. She was awake but severely demented. A specialist in internal medicine testified that Miss Conroy was unable to respond to verbal stimuli, and that she probably no longer possessed any capacity for higher functioning or consciousness. However, her own physician testified that, although Claire Conroy was confused and unaware, "she responds somehow." The testimony at trial also indicated that Miss Conroy was not brain-dead, comatose, or in a chronic vegetative state. As to whether or not she was capable of experiencing pain, the medical testimony was inconclusive.

Both of the doctors who testified at the trial agreed that, if Claire Conroy's nasogastric tube were removed, she would die of dehydration in about a week. They concurred in the opinion that Miss Conroy's death from dehydration would be painful. The specialist in internal medicine testified that, despite the excellent care that Miss Conroy was receiving, she did not have long (perhaps a few months) to live. He considered the nasogastric feeding tube an extraordinary or optional medical treatment, and said that he could recommend that the tube be removed, based upon Miss Conroy's hopeless condition and the possibility that she was suffering in her deteriorated state. On the other hand, Miss Conroy's own physician stated that he did not think it would be acceptable medical practice to remove the tube, and that he was in favor of keeping it in place.

Thomas C. Whittemore was Claire Conroy's only surviving blood relative. He had known her for over fifty years and had continued to visit her regularly, even after her confinement to the nursing home. Based upon his knowledge of Miss Conroy's attitudes, Mr. Whittemore advanced the opinion that if she had been competent she would never have permitted the insertion of the nasogastric tube in the first place.

A Roman Catholic priest and associate professor of Christian Ethics testified that removal of the tube would be ethical and moral, even though the ensuing period up until the patient's death would be painful.

The trial courts decided to permit removal of the tube, finding that Claire Conroy's life had become impossibly and permanently burdensome, and that her intellectual functioning had been permanently reduced to a very primitive level. The judge determined further that removal of the tube would result in death by starvation and dehydration within a few days, and that the death might be painful.

Claire Conroy's guardian *ad litem* appealed and, while that appeal was pending, Miss Conroy died with the nasogastric tube in place. Despite Miss Conroy's death, the Appellate Division of the Superior Court found the issues raised in her case to be of such public importance as to warrant resolution. That court reversed the trial court's judgment, and concluded that withdrawal of the tube would be tantamount to killing her—and not simply letting her die. The court held that such active euthanasia was ethically impermissible. According to the Appellate Division, the right to terminate life-sustaining treatment based on a guardian's judgement was limited to incurable and terminally-ill patients who were brain dead, irreversibly comatose, or vegetative, and who would gain no medical benefit from continued treatment. Alternatively, the court held that a guardian's decision may never be used to withhold nourishment, as opposed to treatment or the attempt to cure a disease, from an incompetent patient who is not comatose, brain-dead, or vegetative, and whose death is not irreversibly imminent.

The New Jersey Supreme Court granted Thomas Whittemore's petition for certification and held *inter alia*:

1. The right of a person to control his own body is a basic societal concept long recognized in the common law.
2. The right to make certain decisions concerning one's body is also protected by the federal constitutional right of privacy.
3. Whether based on common law or constitutional theory, the right to decline life-sustaining medical treatment is not absolute. There are four areas in which the interests of the state may limit the right of a competent person to refuse medical treatment:
   a. *Preserving Life—The Sanctity of All Life*. But this does not prevent a competent person from declining life-sustaining medical treatment for himself.
   b. *Suicide*. Declining life-sustaining medical treatment is not the same as an attempt to commit suicide. Refusing medical intervention merely allows the disease to take its natural course; death would be due to the disease, and not the result of

self-inflicted injury. The distinction is that between self-destruction and self-determination.

c. *Safeguarding the Integrity of the Medical Profession*. This is not threatened by permitting competent patients to refuse life-sustaining medical treatment. Doctors need do no more than advise patients of the risks of foregoing treatment and urge them to accept medical intervention. The patient's right to informed consent is to be respected even when it conflicts with the advice of the doctor or the values of the medical profession as a whole.
d. *Protecting Innocent Third Parties*. Vaccination, minor children and some blood-transfusion cases involve this interest of the state. It is not relevant, however, to the case of the competent adult.

None of these factors applied in the case of Conroy, who was incompetent. Claire Conroy was elderly, formerly competent, a nursing-home resident, awake, conscious, able to interact with her environment to a limited extent, but whose mental and physical functioning had subsequently been severely and permanently impaired, and whose-life expectancy, even with the treatment, was relatively short. Although unable to speak for herself, such a patient retains the right of self-determination even though unable to assert it or to appreciate its application. The goal in such cases should be to determine and effectuate the decision the patient would have made if competent. Therefore, the court held that life-sustaining treatment may be withheld or withdrawn from an imcompetent patient when it is made clear that that particular patient would not wish that treatment under those circumstances. How is this to be determined? The court gives three examples:

1. A Living Will;
2. A Power of Attorney; and
3. Appointment of a Proxy to make the decisions on the patient's behalf if he or she is no longer capable of making them.

Medical evidence must establish that a patient is an elderly, incompetent, nursing-home resident with severe and permanent mental and physical impairment and a life-expectancy of approximately one year or less. Then, the surrogate decision maker must have at least as much medical information upon which to base his decision as a competent patient would require in order to make an informed choice as to whether to accept or reject medical intervention.

If it is not possible to be clearly satisfied as to the patient's intentions, then life-sustaining treatment may *also* be withheld or withdrawn from a patient in Claire Conroy's situation if either of two "best interests" tests is satisfied. One is called the "limited-objective" test; the other is called the "pure-objective" test.

To pass the limited objective test, the situation must meet two conditions. First, there must be some trustworthy evidence that the patient would have refused the treatment. Second, the decision maker must be satisfied that the burdens of the patient's continued life with treatment, outweigh its benefits. Pain becomes the measure. The court says that, to fit into this category of test at all, there needs to be a patient who is suffering, and will continue to suffer, unavoidable pain throughout the expected duration of his or her life. Then, a balance needs to be drawn between two alternatives. Take the pain and suffering expected during the potential life with treatment, and deduct the amount and the duration of pain that the patient would likely experience if the treatment were withdrawn. This is then weighed against the physical pleasure, emotional enjoyment, or intellectual satisfaction that the patient may still be able to derive from life. If the net burden of pain in a prolonged life would clearly seem to be greater, then, under the limited-objective test, termination of treatment for the patient is permitted, provided that he or she had not unequivocally expressed desires to the contrary before becoming incompetent. The essence appears to be that, if the treatment in question merely prolongs the patient's suffering, it should not be commenced or, if already commenced, it may be withdrawn. In the application of this test, the court makes it very clear that medical evidence is essential. The key question seems to be whether or not, given such medical evidence, it can be established that "the treatment would merely prolong the patient's suffering and not provide him with any net benefit." Specific considerations, would include the degree, expected duration, and constancy of pain with and without treatment; the possibility that the pain could be reduced by drugs or other means short of terminating the life-sustaining treatment; the patient's life-expectancy prognosis, level of functioning, degree of humiliation and dependency; and the availability of other treatment options. In addition, the limited-objective test still continues to require "some trustworthy evidence that the patient would have wanted the treatment terminated."

In the absence of clear evidence that the patient would have wanted the treatment terminated, the decision may require the use of the "pure-objective test." This test begins with the same "net-burdens" problem faced in the "limited-objective test." It then goes a step further. For here the court requires that we must determine whether "the recurring, unavoidable, and severe pain of the patient's life with the treatment should be such that the effect of administering life-sustaining treatment would be inhumane." Moreover although we are *required* to determine whether the patient would have wanted the treatment continued, if there is any evidence that this patient had previously expressed a wish to be kept alive no matter what the pain, then the life-sustaining treatment should not be withdrawn.

The court makes a particular effort to cover those questions not specifically decided. One is that no decision is to be made based upon an assessment of the personal worthy or social utility of another's life, or the value that life may hold for others. Thus, the court specifically states that, when the evidence is insufficient to satisfy either the limited-objective or pure-objective standard, the life-sustaining treatment should not be terminated since, the court concludes, this would not further the "best interests" of the patient.

The court goes on to reject some theories previously been put forth by writers on this subject. While stating that the primary focus should be on the patient—his or her desires and potential for experiencing pain and enjoyment—it rejects the following considerations: (1) active conduct vs. passive conduct; (2) any distinction between withholding and withdrawing life-sustaining treatment; (3) any distinction between ordinary treatment and extraordinary treatment; and (4) any distinction between the termination of artificial feedings and the termination of other forms of life—sustaining medical treatment. The court specifically states that there is no significant difference between artificial feedings, artifical breathing, or other mechanical means when the body is no longer able to perform a vital bodily function on its own.

In essence, the court specifically holds that:

> . . . withdrawing or withholding of artificial feeding, like any other medical treatment, would be permissible if there is sufficient proof to satisfy the subjective, limited-objective or pure-objective test. A competent patient has the right to decline any medical treatment, including artificial feeding, and should retain that right when and if he becomes incompetent. In addition, in the case of an incompetent patient who has given little or no trustworthy indication of a intent to decline treatment and for whom it becomes necessary to engage in balancing under the limited-objective or pure-objective test, the pain and invasiveness of an artificial feeding device, and the pain of withdrawing that device, should be treated just like the results of administering or withholding any other medical treatment.

The court compares the decision-making procedure for comatose, vegetative patients suggested in *Quinlan* with the Conroy case, and concludes that it should be different because of the age of the patient, the fact that the patient was in a nursing home, the fact that physicians play a much more limited role in nursing homes than in hospitals, and the fact that nursing homes have peculiar, industry-wide problems less prevalent in hospitals and are therefore not expected to make decisions about a patient's medical care with the same speed that is necessary in hospitals. The process for cases like Claire Conroy's is therefore spelled out to include the following:

1. There must be a judicial determination that the patient is incompetent to make the euthanasia decision for himself, and a guardian is to be appointed for the incompetent patient if one does not already exist. Here the specified question is whether or not the patient is competent to make the particular medical treatment decision at issue at the time. Unless and until he or she is adjudicated to be incompetent in this sense, he or she must be considered competent. In order to guide future decision makers, the definition of competence is stated in the alternative. A patient may be considered incompetent in this sense if he or she lacks the ability to understand the information conveyed, to evaluate the options, or to communicate a decision. Here, the court will require medical evidence bearing on these capabilities. This evidence must be furnished to a court by at least two doctors, with expertise in relevant fields, who have personally examined the patient; and the court must be satisfied, by clear and convincing evidence,

that the patient does not have, and will not regain, the capacity to make the decision for himself. The court stresses the fact that the test of competence deals specifically with the particular medical treatment decision, and that competence of other sorts, such as the ability to "govern" one's self and manage one's other affairs, does not necessarily apply. If a guardian has already been appointed for this patient for some other reason, the court will still investigate whether or not the patient can make the particular medical decision in question.

2. These proceedings may be commenced by any person who believes that withholding or withdrawing life-sustaining treatment would effectuate an incompetent patient's wishes, or would be in his "best interests." Such a person must notify the Office of the Ombudsman. Any person who believes the contrary should also report such information to the Ombudsman.
3. The Ombudsman must treat every notification as a possible "abuse" and is required to investigate the situation and report it within 24 hours to the Commissioner of Human Services and to any other government agency that regulates or operates the facility.
4. Evidence must then be presented as to the patient's condition by the attending physician and nurses. Two other physicians, unaffiliated with the nursing-home and with the attending physician, should then be appointed to confirm the patient's medical condition and prognosis. The court recommends that the Ombudsman exercise his discretionary authority to appoint the physicians as provided for in the statute.
5. Provided that the two physicians supply the necessary medical foundation, the guardian, with the concurrence of the attending physician, may withhold or withdraw life-sustaining medical treatment if he or she believes, in good faith, based upon the medical evidence and any evidence of the patient's wishes, that it is clear that the requirements of either the subjective, limited-objective, or pure-objective tests have been satisfied. However, the Ombudsman must concur in that decision.
6. Finally, if either the limited objective or pure-objective test is being used, the family—that is, the patient's spouse, parents, and children (or, in their absence, the patient's next of kin, if any)—must also concur in the decision to withhold or withdraw life-sustaining treatment.

The involvement of the court in this procedure is limited to the determination of incompetency of the patient, as described above, and the appointment of a guardian. Thereafter, it is up to the guardian to resolve the issues and make the ultimate decision, applying those standards described and set forth by the court.

In conclusion, the court specifically mentions certain cases to which these decisions do not necessarily apply: the severely deformed newborn, the never-competent adult suffering from a painful and debilitating illness, and the mentally alert quadriplegic who has given up on life.

A special additional opinion was rendered by Justice Handler, who concurred in part, and dissented in part. Although his opinion is not considered binding, some of his comments should be considered.

Justice Handler is uncomfortable with the fact that the majority opinion focuses on pain as the critical factor, so that the presence of significant pain in effect becomes the sole measure of a person's best interests. It was his feeling that "pain" eclipses a whole cluster of other human values that have a proper place in the subtle process of thought that will ultimately determine how life should end. The exclusive-pain criterion denies relief to that class of people who, at the very end of life, might strongly disapprove of an artificially extended existence in spite of the absence of any pain. It was his feeling that the standard should consist of an array of medically established factors evaluated by the decision maker, both singly and collectively, to reach a balance. Such a test should be applied only when the person is terminally ill, facing imminent death, permanently unconscious or comatose, and suffering from the irreparable failure of at least one major and essential bodily organ or system.

Special problems have arisen when the question of withdrawal of hydration and nutrition is presented. If the patient is competent, it has been allowed. One example is the case of Beverly Requena, which was decided in New Jersey by a trial court in September, 1986. She was a 55-year-old woman dying of amyotrophic lateral sclerosis (ALS) or "Lou Gehrig's Disease." While mentally alert, she made an informed decision to exercise her right to die by requesting that when, as her diseased progressed, she lost her ability to swallow, she did not wish to be fed by a nasogastric tube or "other artificial device." This was acknowledged, respected, and approved by the Appellate Division of the New Jersey Superior Court even though the hospital's policy and staff preference were to the contrary.

The same thing occurred true in June, 1986, when a trial court in Ocean County considered a case entitled, *In the Matter of Kathleen Farrell*, 212 NJ Super 294, 514 A2d. 1342. In that case, Kathleen Farrell, a 37-year-old married woman with two sons, ages 16 and 14, was suffering from ALS, and was on a respirator. Her husband made an application to the court to be appointed special medical guardian for his wife, with the added request that he be given express permission to remove the respirator. The court was convinced that the patient was competent and wished to terminate the treatment, even knowing that it would most likely cause her death. The court, in rendering the specific decision, did not state that the guardian had the right to carry out the wishes of his wife, since this would imply that he need not exercise that right if he should change his mind. Instead, the words of the Judgment were such that it was tantamount to an Order to remove the respirator. However, it is interesting to question the court's use of the additional words "with the advice of her treating physician." Did this mean that, if the treating physician had changed his advice before the respirator was removed, the guardian would no longer have the protection of the Order of the court contained in its final ruling, namely, that in the removal of the respirator neither the physician nor any other person involved could be held criminally or civilly responsible? The final determination was in accord with the *Quinlan* decision, which stated, "the ensuing death would not be homicide, but rather expiration from existing natural causes. Secondly, even if it were to be regarded as homicide, it would not be unlawful." The *Quinlan* court added that there is a "real and determinative distinction between the unlawful taking of the life of another and the ending of artificial life support systems as a matter of self-determination.'' The court clearly established that the exercise of this constitutional right is protected from criminal prosecution, which ''extends to third parties whose action is necessary to effectuate the exercise of that right.''

On June 24, 1987, the New Jersey Supreme Court rendered decisions in three companion cases. One was the *Farrell* case referred to above, another was *In re Peter*, and the third was *In re Jobes*. In the *Farrell* decision, the court reaffirmed that a patient's right to refuse medical treatment, even at the risk of personal injury or death, is protected both by common law and by Federal and State Constitutional right to privacy. If a patient is mentally competent and living at home and requests the discontinuance of life-sustaining medical treatment, there is a specific procedure which must be followed. The first step is an assessment of the mental competence of the patient. If the requirement of competence is met with, the second step is confirmation that the patient is properly informed about his or her prognosis, the alternative treatments available, and the risks involved in the withdrawal of life-sustaining treatment. That all of these requirements have been met with must be based upon the findings of two non-attending physicians who have examined the patient at home. If this procedure is followed, there is no need for an application to a court, and judicial participation is not necessary. These rules apply only to the competent, informed patient at home who decides to refuse medical treatment.

The *Peter* case involved a permanently unconscious adult in a nursing home who, unlike Claire Conroy, was not expected to die within a year. The patient's condition was held to render the life expectancy test inappropriate. Since the patient could not contribute to decision-making, the case became a surrogate-refusal-of-treatment case and the ''subjective'' test became applicable. The patient's wishes were considered controlling. Life-sustaining treatment can be foregone when there is ''clear and convincing'' proof that the patient would, if competent, decline treatment. The court commented that a living will or a durable power of attorney would be the best substitute evidence of a patient's wishes. Since New Jersey has a statute creating the position known as ''Ombudsman,'' the role of that office in a case of this kind needed to be clarified. The New Jersey Supreme Court has stated that surrogate-decision makers are required to inform the Office of the Ombudsman that a decision to withhold or withdraw treatment has been made. The Ombudsman must secure two independent medical opinions to confirm the patient's irreversible condition, the medical alternatives available, the risks involved, and the likely outcome if treatment is discontinued. If there is ''clear and convincing evidence'' that the patient has designated a family member or ''close friend'' to make surrogate medical decisions, upon receipt of the two medical confirmations, the Ombudsman should defer decisions about life support to that person. If there is no designated person, the Ombudsman must consult with the health-care providers to ascertain whether there is a ''close caring family member'' (normally a spouse, parent, adult child or sibling) who will be willing and able to make such decisions. If there is, the Ombudsman should defer decisions about life support to that person. Judicial review of a surrogate decision is unnecessary unless a conflict arises among the surrogate decision-maker, the family, the physician and the Ombudsman. Guardians must be appointed for a patient for whom there is no person who can adequately represent the patient's interests. Close friends cannot make surrogate decisions on a patient's behalf unless the patient has specifically designated them in that role. The *Peter* case therefore clarifies procedures for foregoing life support for an elderly, incompetent nursing home patient in a persistent vegetative state, emphasizing the role of patients' surrogates, and decreasing the role of the Ombudsman and the Courts. This decision is the first of its kind in the United States which takes a definite position as to the weight to be given to the appointment of a proxy by a patient to deal with matters of health-care when the patient is unable to do so himself or herself. The decision is also important because it takes a clear position that artificial feeding is a type of medical treatment which can be withdrawn, and if a patient dies subsequent to such a withdrawal, the cause of death is the underlying disease, and not the withdrawal of artificial feeding.

The third companion case was *In re Jobes*. Nancy Jobes was an adult nursing home patient in a persistent vegetative state who was under the age of sixty. If she had been sixty or over, the Office of the Ombudsman would have been a required participant. The question was whether or not artificial feeding, as a form of medical treatment, could be terminated. The court responded by stating that its role was to establish criteria respecting the right of self-determination while protecting incompetent patients. The court found that the patient's family could use its substituted judgment to effectuate as much as possible the decision which the patient would have made if competent. If there are no close family members and the patient has not left "clear and convincing evidence" that he or she intended another relative or non-relative friend to make decisions for him or her, then a guardian should be appointed by the court. Once we have either the close family member, the appointed friend, or a guardian, a specific procedure must be followed. The decision maker must secure statements from at least two independent physicians knowledgeable in neurology, as well as from the attending physician, if there is one, declaring that the patient is in a persistent vegetative state and that there is no reasonable possibility that the patient will ever return to a cognitive, sapient state.

The incompetent patient who has never expressed his or her desires continues to be a problem. *In the Matter of George Clark*, decided April 7, 1986, at 210 NJ Super 548, 510 A2d. 136, a special application needed to be made to the court. The patient's condition was not the same as in the *Quinlan* model, and the patient was not in a nursing home so *Conroy* could not be applied. Here the court weighed the burden of life with an enterostomy as compared to the benefit of the indefinite life expectancy of a patient with organic brain damage, a low cognitive level, severe neurological and medical conditions, but in neither a vegetative or comatose state. Since the family, the treating and consulting physicians, and the hospital's Optimal Care Committee could not agree, the court chose in favor of ordering the procedure.

In *In the Matter of Elizabeth Visbeck*, Superior Court of New Jersey, Chancery Division, Morris County, Docket No. P–29–86E, in an Opinion by Hon. Reginald Stanton, 210 NJ Super 527, issued on February 4, 1986, the question presented was whether a feeding tube should be surgically implanted in the stomach of a 90-year-old patient who had suffered a severe disabling stroke. Without the feeding tube, the patient would suffer death from dehydration and starvation. With the tube, the nutritional needs of the patient would be fully met, although she would remain permanently in a very poor physical and mental condition. The court decided that the feeding tube should be implanted, and in doing so, considered the following:

1. This was the only effective way to meet the patient's nutritional needs.
2. The surgical procedure involved was simple and could be performed under local anesthetic.
3. The patient had some appreciable awareness of her surroundings and some meaningful capacity to react to them.
4. Nurses testified that they occasionally heard the patient speak distinct words or phrases, and her son testified that, as recently as a few days before, the patient had given coherent answers to certain questions.
5. The patient was not *in* pain, although she was capable of feeling pain.
6. There was no evidence at all bearing on what the patient would have decided under the circumstances now confronting her.
7. The ongoing use of the tube would not be uncomfortable for the patient.
8. The health-care providers saw positive value to the feeding, and the court-appointed guardian agreed.

The conclusion to implant the tube was reached even though the medical evidence revealed that the patient suffered from congestive heart failure; still had fibrillation problems despite the presence of a pacemaker; had received massive damage to the right side of her brain; was paralyzed on the left side of her body; was nonambulatory, basically noncommunicative, and unable to swallow; and had no control of bowel or bladder function. Moreover, it was made despite the fact that none of these conditions were likely to improve in any significant way. The medical testimony clearly stated that she probably would not live more than a few months even if all of her needs for nourishment were met. The judgement nevertheless reserved for the court the opportunity to review the matter if changes in the patient's mental or physical condition occurred, or if there was a significant adverse reaction to the tube or to feeding through it.

The court gave some insight into what might be considered in a further application by stating the following:

There is a troublesome aspect to feeding tube cases which I think deserves some thought. Although respect for life is one of our most worthy characteristics, and although the instinct to keep living is one of our strongest drives, there comes a time when each of us must die. Delaying that time by active medical treatment and by other active means makes sense so long as there is some minimally acceptable quality to the life which is prolonged. There comes some point at which virtually every reasonble person would call a halt to treatment. There is some point at which, in a very real sense, a person is supposed to die. I think that when massive and irreversible loss of the higher brain functions is followed by the permanent loss of ability to swallow, we may be dealing with a natural and fitting closing-down of the total human organism. I think that artificial feeding and other forms of active treatment are mandatory until we are sure that we are dealing with massive and irreversible loss of the higher brain functions. However, once we are sure that we are dealing with a massive and irreversible loss of the higher brain functions, I suggest that true decency might lead us to be very cautious about interfering with the natural closing down of the human body.

In the closing paragraphs of the opinion, the judge stated that certain conditions "might justify withdrawal of the tube in the near future or in the more distant future," but did not say that it would require a further application to the court. Instead, in the earlier part of the opinion the court stated that "so long as Elizabeth Visbeck is a patient at Chilton Memorial Hospital or any other hospital, removal of the tube may not occur without agreement of the prognosis committee of the hospital." A question remains as to whether or not the court was stating that the prognosis committee had the power to make the decision, or whether such agreement was a prerequisite to further application to the court. The specific words chosen seem to be quite careful and significant. It appears that the court was thinking in terms of the *Quinlan* case, where such authority was given to the prognosis committee acting together with the family and the attending physician without any need to return to court as long as it appeared that there was no likelihood the patient would return to a cognitive sapient state.

While we await furuther guidance from the New Jersey Supreme Court or, hopefully, from the New Jersey Legislature, the status of the New Jersey Law as of January 1987 appears to be:

1. The competent patient's decision controls. (Apparently this refers to termination, not prolongation of care. "Econo-ethics" needs to come out of gestation as third parties cut off benefits and force discharges in spite of the contrary feelings of providers and/or patients.)
2. The incompetent patient is dealt with differently in each setting.
   A. The incompetent patient in a nursing home is treated very specially. This is due to New Jersey's historical problems with such facilities. If all of the conditions set forth in *Conroy* can be met, then and only then can the patient be terminated.
   B. The incompetent patient in a hospital may fall into many different categories, only some of which have received attention. In cases like *Quinlan, Visbeck*, and *Clark*, we have patients whose prognosis as to life expectancy is either "unknown," "indefinite," or "short," without regard to a finding of "vegetative state." In

Visbeck and *Clark*, the court found sufficient probable benefit to be achieved from treatment to warrant treatment continuity or intervention. Even a finding of medical uncertainty as to possible benefit was sufficient. It would appear to then follow that, in the absence of such a finding, such a patient could be terminated without civil or criminal responsibility.

C. The incompetent patient at home has not as yet received special legal attention.

In the middle of 1986, New Jersey passed a statute creating the New Jersey Commission on Legal and Ethical Problems in the Delivery of Health Care. The Commission is charged with studying the issues considered above, as well as related ones such as sterilization, living wills, medical power of attorney, determination of death, and so forth. The commission's first report is due at the end of 1988. If the legislature has not acted before then, perhaps some guidance will be forthcoming from the commission. In the interim, health care providers are at legal risk, and consumers are at life risk.

The *New Jersey Law Journal*, which is considered to be the voice of the members of the bar of the state of New Jersey, published an editorial on July 10, 1986, wherein it was stated that "because of the great advances in medical technology, perhaps society should begin to consider euthanasia as acceptable in some circumstances." The article went on to say, "It is unfortunate that the judicial system must resolve these issues without any guidelines established by the citizens of the state of New Jersey."

Perhaps it is appropriate to reconsider a presentation made by the author at the annual meeting of the Medical Society of New Jersey on May 16, 1981, later published in *The Journal of the Medical Society of New Jersey*, November, 1981, Vol. 78, No. 12, pp. 812–5, and entitled "Euthanasia: Where Are We? Where Are We Going?" This author, after acknowledging the primacy of patient autonomy when it could be determined, acknowledged that in other situations the concept of "quality of life" is the major consideration in determining whether or not to terminate life-support systems for the incompetent patient whose desires are otherwise indeterminable.

Index

www.ingramcontent.com/pod-product-compliance
Ingram Content Group UK Ltd.
Pitfield, Milton Keynes, MK11 3LW, UK
UKHW020811290926
15470UKWH00003B/1088

9 780275 92595